Listening in the Silence,
Seeing in the Dark

Ruthann Knechel Johansen

Listening in the Silence, Seeing in the Dark

Reconstructing Life
after Brain Injury

UNIVERSITY OF CALIFORNIA PRESS

Berkeley   Los Angeles   London

University of California Press
Berkeley and Los Angeles, California

University of California Press, Ltd.
London, England

Library of Congress Cataloging-in-Publication Data

Johansen, Ruthann Knechel, 1942–.
    Listening in the silence, seeing in the dark : reconstructing life after brain injury / Ruthann Knechel Johansen.
        p.   cm.
    Includes bibliographical references and index.
    ISBN 0-520-23114-7 (cloth : alk. paper).
    1. Johansen, Erik, 1969– —Health.   2. Brain—Wounds and injuries—Patients—Biography.   3. Brain—Wounds and injuries—Patients—Rehabilitation.   4. Brain—Wounds and injuries—Patients—Family relationships.   5. Bibliotherapy.   6. Storytelling—Therapeutic use.   7. Parents of children with disabilities.   I. Title.
RJ496.B7 J65   2002
362.1'97481044'092—dc21   2001027681
                                                                    [B]

Manufactured in the United States of America

10   09   08   07   06   05   04   03   02
10   9   8   7   6   5   4   3   2   1

The paper used in this publication is both acid-free and totally chlorine-free (TCF). It meets the minimum requirements of ANSI/NISO Z39.48-1992 (R 1997) (*Permanence of Paper*).

For
Erik, Sonia, Robert,
and all who wait in silence

Giving birth and nourishing,
having without possessing,
acting with no expectations,
leading and not trying to control:
this is the supreme virtue.

Tao te Ching

Vision begins to happen in such a life
as if a woman quietly walked away
from the argument and jargon in a room
and sitting down in the kitchen, began turning in her lap
bits of yarn, calico, and velvet scraps,
laying them out absently on the scrubbed boards
in the lamplight . . .
and skeins of milkweed from the nearest meadow—
original domestic silk, the finest findings—
and the darkblue petal of the petunia,
and the dry darkbrown lace of seaweed;
. . . .
Such a composition has nothing to do with eternity,
the striving for greatness, brilliance—
only with the musing of a mind
one with her body, experienced fingers quietly pushing
dark against bright, silk against roughness,
pulling the tenets of a life together
with no mere will to mastery,
only care for the many-lived, unending
forms in which she finds herself,
becoming now the sherd of broken glass
slicing light in a corner, dangerous
to flesh, now the plentiful, soft leaf
that wrapped round the throbbing finger, soothes the wound;
and now the stone foundation, rockshelf further
forming underneath everything that grows.

Adrienne Rich, "Transcendental Etude"

Contents

Introduction

This book is about silence
to find one's way
Here I lay side by side
of my young son's life story
to bridge the gap between
to translate my *knowing*
Walking with our son through
back toward a radically revised life
to experiment with
the loss of consciousness
through telling.
Breaking apart the self
and integrated,
reveals the inchoate,
On the threshold
and language
Stripped of his ability
and self-representation

and darkness and the struggle
toward the light.
the shattered fragments
and my dependence on metaphors
continuity and discontinuity,
experience into *telling*.
the shadows of nonbeing and
forces this story
fashioning his *not knowing*—
and memory—into *knowing*
and retelling.
that has appeared coherent
traumatic brain injury
hidden from our sight.
between silence
lies the obliterated self.
for self-regard
his condition opens a crack

This is a story of how the already born, when afflicted with traumatic brain injury, must be reborn, taking a far more arduous journey into life. In the second birth, such individuals face greater challenges with diminished abilities. Though this is a book I wish I would never have had the knowledge to write, it is also a book I wish I would have had as a parent waiting through the long, starless nights of coma or later searching in vain for reliable markings along the path back into life.

In the spring of 1985, our bright, handsome, energetic fifteen-year-old son suffered a traumatic brain injury, thrusting him and us as his family into a chaotic, mysterious space between being and nonbeing. When severe injury assaulted our son's brain and central nervous system, his self no longer functioned in customary ways: motor activity, sensation, and cognition stopped, and all "languages" that support these capacities were temporarily useless. His story appeared to stop. Along with shock and anguish, questions poured out of me. Will he live? Will he ever regain consciousness? And if consciousness, at what level of capability? Can he know himself or be known to others without speaking? Who will speak for Erik? In this void or psychic-liminal space, which is always a nightmarish region for the injured and his or her family, I desperately wondered how our son might become a self a second time or navigate this radical breach in his developing life story. What follows is my description of that silent, empty space with our son and of his struggle to live and to climb back into language and story.

Because traumatic brain injury has reached near epidemic proportions in the United States and the industrialized world, and because the cost of treating brain injury and rehabilitating its victims continues to soar, none of us is untouched. Though this is the story of one young man, I write to bear witness for all who struggle courageously, though often invisibly, to restore their lives following traumatic brain injury. As I write, I have been attended particularly by the felt presence of Neil, Danny, Todd, Caroline, Doug, Don, Tracy, Janet, and David. Each of these people—varying in age from fourteen to the forties, living in different parts of the United States and outside it, and working to live fully despite the effects of brain injuries—has directly shared his or her experience of acquired brain injury with me or, in the silence inflicted by injury, has left a visible imprint in my mind. Their struggles to recompose their own lives run quietly beneath the surface of the story I know best.

The attempt to portray Erik's process of personal reconstruction, which takes place on many levels at once, requires this book to move on more than one level. First, the process includes the interior territory of Erik's brain and body, of which I can only report from my observations and engagement with the outward manifestations of an inner, invisible story line. Second, my husband, my daughter, and I all had unique reactions to Erik and his injuries and responded to him differently, each making separate, though entwined, stories from the experience. Each parsed the facts individually as we resisted wrong or partial stories and tried to invite a son and brother to second life. Third, every treatment protocol, each doctor, therapist, educator, and friend extended a link in a long chain of being for Erik to grasp.

Just as working with a family member who has suffered a traumatic brain injury demands ceaseless experimentation to help him or her reassemble his or her shattered pieces, so attempting to bear witness to the process of reorganizing a life has required the invention of a form to convey the experience. This is not a book of head injury resources or prescriptions, nor is it simply a medical biography. It is, rather, a meditation, with and through stories, about the dialogical character of our biological, psychological, and social lives made visible in the loss of consciousness and language and through shattered dreams. Using my consciousness to describe the life of our unconscious son, to feel and participate in the pain of his undoing, and to reflect on his reconstruction, I invite multiple audiences—families, medical and rehabilitation professionals, insurance brokers, lawyers, educators, and indeed an entire society in which the preoccupation with being author and lead character of our individual stories always obscures our relational interdependence—to linger and perhaps to learn on the threshold between continuity and discontinuity, death and life.

The Impact of Vulnerability

I am a teacher of stories.
Stories ancient and mythic.
Stories purportedly factual and historical.
And stories that are fictitious, made
in the imagination and shaped
and reshaped by tellers.
I am also a mother.
One who has read and told stories.
One who has listened to
and encouraged stories from my children.

In 1985 my husband Robert and I were rearing twelve-year-old Sonia and fifteen-year-old Erik in Princeton Junction, a New Jersey suburban community, with the attendant pressures and opportunities typical of professional suburban commuter families. Robert commuted to New York City three days a week to his office at a research institute; on Tuesdays and Thursdays I traveled south to teach American literature at Stockton State College.

One October evening in 1984 my son approached me. "I need to write a poem. Well, actually two poems for English class tomorrow. One must tell a story, and the other can create an image." Sensing Erik's impatience with an assignment falling outside his interest in math and computers, I asked, "Any other guidelines?" I was stalling for time, thinking how to surmount his frustration and to entice him into this wonderful linguistic territory. "No models?" I asked. Growing more visibly restless, he said "Nope" in a tone that only slightly concealed a "how many times must I tell you?" attitude. "I get it," I said; "this is an assignment that simply throws you out into the deep water, where you'll sink or swim." "Yeah, I guess," was all he said.

Scenes similar to this typically occur in homes where teens reside. Often they end here, with parent and child parting company, each feeling a bit at sea. This particular evening, however, we pursued our conversation despite the anxiety these unknown waters produced. Soon we were talking about the song lyrics of his favorite musicians—Phil Collins, Yes, Genesis. We considered the stories their songs tell. Then I asked if he had ideas about a story he wanted to tell. His ideas were broad and abstract: about love, about sadness. I thought of Shakespeare's sonnets. We read a few and talked about their stories. About the emotions and the images used to convey emotions. About compression of language. About metaphors and rhythm in language.

Then John Donne's "A Valediction Forbidding Mourning" popped into my mind. Perhaps the regular rhythmic pattern in which it relates its story would provide a structural framework for Erik's attempts at poetic storytelling. We read the first stanza.

A VALEDICTION FORBIDDING MOURNING

As virtuous men pass mildly away,
And whisper to their souls to go,
Whilst some of their sad friends do say,
"Now his breath goes," and some say "No";

We read on, he speaking one stanza, then I the next, on throughout the poem, letting the rhythm seep into his ears and mind. We continued on through the last four stanzas, attending to the sounds and images. Many years later memory brought that night of reading and the prophetic power of the closing stanzas to my full consciousness.

> Our two souls therefore, which are one,
> Though I must go, endure not yet
> A breach, but an expansion,
> Like gold to airy thinness beat.
>
> If they be two, they are two so
> As stiff twin compasses are two,
> Thy soul, the fixed foot, makes no show
> To move, but doth, if th' other do.
>
> And though it in the centre sit,
> Yet when the other far doth roam,
> It leans and hearkens after it,
> And grows erect as that comes home.
>
> Such wilt thou be to me, who must
> Like th' other foot, obliquely run,
> Thy firmness makes my circle just,
> And makes me end where I begun.

The regular meter seemed to offer Erik a life preserver for the choppy waters of poem-making, and, fortunately, the subject captured his attention. He began to link his abstractions of love and sadness to the concrete physical form and his perception of his maternal grandmother. He compared Grandma K's worsening osteoporosis and stoic silence in an environment of criticism and denial to Donne's advice to make no noise, to shed no tears nor sigh. Together, back and forth, we tossed out images and possible lines until, ready to launch out on his own, Erik began to piece together his poem born of imitation and conversation.

When he brought the finished product to me we both were pleased. My son's satisfaction derived largely from completing an assignment before midnight and gaining a superficial appreciation of poetic form. Mine came from recognizing in this exchange the ways that language permits us to narrate stories and, indeed, becomes the bricks with which we construct our own life habitations. It was impossible on that autumn evening to anticipate the events that lay ahead and the ways our poem-making from Donne's metaphor in "Valediction" would become incarnated for Erik and our family. As Donne's poem had become the "fixed foot" for Erik's poem-making, so our bodies and souls would be required to "in the centre sit" as Erik's roamed afar.

By the end of his sophomore year, which had begun with the poem-making, Erik was completing courses in architecture, calculus, Bible, ancient history, French, and physics in addition to English. He had traded in piano and cello lessons for playing baseball and was advancing through the beginning belts of karate with enthusiasm and adeptness. He had taken the PSAT and received scores that put him on the mailing lists of the country's finest colleges. Because of his interest in computers and programming, he resourcefully had written a résumé, circulated it, and, much to our surprise, landed a summer job at a local computer store.

Almost every Sunday morning our family attended worship at the Society of Friends Meeting. Erik and Sonia had participated in the religious education classes, and my husband and I had contributed to the religious education program, for about six years. The Young Friends, a group of high school youth, had planned a one-day canoe trip for the last Sunday in May 1985, only a few weeks before the end of school for our children. Erik waffled all Saturday evening about participating; he wanted to take a school friend with him, but he couldn't reach the youth adviser to check whether there would be sufficient canoe space for a visitor. Finally on Sunday morning, with his father's encouragement, he decided to join the group without his friend. He made his bag lunch and jauntily said good-bye in the kitchen. I reminded him to call us if he discovered he wouldn't be home in time to join us for an evening picnic with a group of family friends. Robert drove him to the meeting house and bade the zestful two-car group farewell, after ensuring that Erik would ride in the adult adviser's car.

Later on that gloriously clear May morning Sonia, Robert, and I returned to Meeting. During the last five minutes of the worship a member rose and delivered this short message: "None of us knows how long he will live." Shattering the silence, these few words disturbed me, turning my peaceful meditation into brief but uneasy reflection. Then the rise of Meeting lulled me back into the customary complacencies of enjoying the weather and our friends.

After worship Robert and Sonia went home, but I remained at the meeting house for a committee meeting. My own academic year had just ended, and I was looking forward to cleaning the large bucket of strawberries that Sonia and I had picked the day before. Shortly after the meeting began it was interrupted by a telephone call from Kessler Hospital in Hammonton, New Jersey, two hours south of Princeton. The caller was trying to locate some family member of an injured party. I was the only one on the committee who knew anything about the Young Friends' canoe trip, so I took the call, knowing only that there had been an accident apparently involving our young people.

Even as I write, fourteen years later, I feel my pulse quicken and adrenaline pump through my body. Within seconds I was informed that *our* son was injured, that hospital personnel were seeking permission to care for him, and that I should come as quickly as possible. I had the presence of mind to ask if Erik was conscious; the caller said only that she had not seen him but thought that he had been banged around pretty badly.

Incredulous and terrified, I desperately tried to hang on to any thread of hope that he would be all right. She hadn't said he was unconscious, I argued with myself, so why should I imagine something worse than might be? I tried to concentrate on the directions to the hospital the caller was giving me, staggering mentally between collapse and refusal to believe. I almost missed her closing words. "I think you should bring someone with you." When I hung up the phone it was 12:30 P.M., but it might as easily have been 5:00 A.M., or 9:00 P.M. tomorrow, or in another life-time. I felt no breeze and heard no birds. Totally unaware that two hours away the words "survival in question" were being written in a hospital admissions report, I walked past the meeting house cemetery to the car and began to fight unconsciously for my son's life.

A rocklike silence rose in me as friends drove me home to break the news to Robert and Sonia. Into that silence rushed questions, questions like "Where was the youth adviser in whose car Erik had been riding when they left the meeting house?" and "Why didn't he call us?" I tried to sub-due catastrophic mental images of death and severely mangled bodies of the entire canoe party. When that failed, I took a thread of my fear, stretched it as far as I could away from what was happening, and emotion-ally climbed onto it to avoid being devoured by terror. Within a few fran-tic minutes of my saying, "Erik is hurt," the three of us were on the road, with our close friend Mike driving us the two hours to Hammonton.

As we rode on the highways I used twice each week to commute between my home and Stockton College, the bulwark of silence within me grew. Riding beside Mike in the front seat, my husband expressed his fear, anguish, and grief visibly and audibly: "Oh, God, I shouldn't have told him to go. . . . This is awful. . . . It's all my fault." Sonia and I sat close together in the back seat; eventually she laid her head in my lap, moving between dreadful waiting and the oblivion of sleep. Out of the silence and without conscious bidding, words from a hymn I had played and sung in church as a child began to circle repetitively in my head: "My hope is built on nothing less than Jesus Christ my righteousness . . . on Christ the solid rock I stand, all other ground is sinking sand. . . ." Over and over, mantralike, "on Christ the solid rock I stand" bore me to our injured son.

At the hospital we were met by Richard Weeder, the Young Friends' adviser, who was a surgeon himself, and the emergency room physician. Both tried to be reassuring, describing for us everything that had already been done for Erik. Yes, he was unconscious, for he had received sig-nificant blows to the head, but the paramedics had arrived within minutes of the accident. They had started oxygen even as the Jaws of Life worked to extricate him from the car. They had pumped particles of food, inhaled during the impact, from his lungs. They had checked for signs of internal bleeding and injury. They had already taken a CT scan, which looked ambiguous—they couldn't tell how much the brain stem might have been affected. He had no major external lacerations or broken bones except for the left clavicle. I listened stoically to this important recital of services rendered, but all I wanted was to see our son.

Finally we were allowed in. I proceeded on rubbery legs and with a pounding heart through two sets of double doors. I was not prepared to see Erik, bone of my bone and flesh of my flesh, looking physically much as he had when we had said good-bye six hours earlier. Some small cuts on his face had been cleaned up. My whole being inwardly leapt to gather his motionless and silent form into my arms. As he lay in a half-reclining position with a tube in his nose and other lines attaching him to monitors and a respirator, we talked to him, telling him that we were there and would stay with him; we touched him, trying physically and verbally to convey our love. We called to him, asking him gently if he could hear us, trying to reassure him and ourselves. I kept hoping that familiar voices would rouse him, as they always do in the movies. He made no response even to strong pinches of his skin and the pulling of hairs on his legs. While we stood by him the attending physician lifted Erik's eyelids to check his pupils. What I saw registered in those brown eyes was utter terror, not unlike the expression I'd once seen on the face of an injured deer that had been hit by an automobile. How could I reach the being behind those eyes?

Though he had first told us that Kessler Hospital had everything Erik would need, the physician now recommended that we move Erik to a hospital better equipped and staffed to handle traumatic injuries. Since this was a holiday weekend, the Kessler units were short staffed. Cooper Hospital in Camden was the closest with a specialized trauma unit. Later that evening, I wondered why Erik had not been taken there originally. Was it because his survival was in question? Or was it that initially no one knew the severity of his injuries and could only begin to speculate about them as the hours passed? Confronted with a world of medical crisis wholly new to us and committed to securing the best care we could for our son, we relied heavily on the advice of the hospital doctor, our doctor-friend Richard, and our own instincts. We decided to move Erik to Camden and asked if one of us might accompany Erik in the ambulance. My husband and I were refused permission, but Dr. Weeder was allowed to join the transport. That was our small effort not to leave Erik comfortless in this threatening terrain.

As we drove over unfamiliar roads, trailing several miles behind the ambulance, the physical gulf widened between us and our son. Not only was he unconscious and incapable of communicating; now also he had become the ward of medical guardians. When he arrived at Cooper Hospital he was whisked into examination. The trauma physicians on duty detected internal bleeding, which had not been discovered previously, and informed us that surgery was necessary. A severe impact, one in which the human body becomes a projectile, often damages the spleen, liver, kidneys, and even the lungs and heart. The doctor explained that a seriously damaged spleen can be removed if necessary without unduly endangering the patient's life. Seven hours into this nightmarish ordeal we again were required to make a decision for which the outcome could not be assured. We signed the appropriate papers and moved to the trauma unit waiting area. Weary and tense, Robert and I sat numbly in a stream of grief rising steadily. After three hours the doctors reported that Erik's spleen had been lacerated but was repairable. To our great relief and gratitude his other organs seemed not to be in jeopardy, though the condition of his brain remained uncertain.

Night fell as nurses completed postoperative routines and settled Erik, armed with multiple mechanical monitors, into a curtained cubicle in the trauma unit. Night brought other darknesses. It was obvious that we would not take Erik home with us; indeed, we ourselves would not go home that night or for many subsequent nights. But our friends could not stay. And what about Sonia? What was best for her? Slowly we were forced to consider the "ordinary" world of school and jobs, of a missed picnic, of our extended families half a continent away, and of Erik's friends. We made the fewest heartbreaking calls we could, soliciting hope for Erik in this dark hour in which his life dangled uncertainly before our eyes. We decided to wrap Sonia in our friends' love and send her home with them for the night. They would return the next day, Memorial Day.

By the time Erik's surgery was finished all the people who had been in the waiting area earlier had disappeared. We did not realize that visits in the trauma unit were limited to two hours per day, one hour in the late morning and one hour in the early evening. The hospital staff did not discourage us from staying in the waiting room the first night and told us that we could see him once each hour. Having had previous exposure to pediatric intensive care units, where brief visits once an hour were the norm, I did not think to question whether this was a standard practice or a courtesy accommodation extended to families in the initial throes of shock. Did the hospital staff perhaps offer this opportunity because they were not too busy? Or was it because Erik's life hung delicately in the balance that first night?

That night Robert and I, together or singly, sat by Erik's inert form, listening to the blips and beeps of his machine-generated breathing, watching his body functions represented through electronic signs. It was as if we had suddenly been transported into a foreign country, the language, signs, and symbols of which we had little understanding. Our son was absolutely helpless in this new world. We could and did ask questions about the procedures performed on him, about the normal ranges for heartbeat, respiration, and blood pressure, about this totally new phenomenon of intracranial pressure following a traumatic blow to the head. We were curious, intelligent, and generally informed, and we knew instinctively that we would assist our vulnerable son.

What did we expect that first night? I cannot now remember expecting anything, for all our physical energy and mental attention were poured into navigating in this nightmarish set of circumstances that we had never imagined for ourselves or our children. Through bizarre, chance events on a rare day in May we joined the vast company of earth's people who are forced to struggle merely to survive. I am sure that every minute I hoped Erik would open his eyes, rejoin us in consciousness, and allow us to leave the fear that bound us.

Some time after midnight we began to take turns trying to sleep, wrapped in hospital blankets on vinyl chairs pushed together to hold our legs and feet. At some level, the lack of response from Erik's body to painful stimuli and the pessimistic tone of doctors' voices when they reported that no one could predict the outcome of Erik's injuries hinted that our sojourn in this foreign world of medical crisis might end abruptly, a hint I missed as we began a defiant watch. As one of us slept fitfully in hour-long shifts, waiting for some flicker of hope, the other sat by Erik, stroking him, speaking gently to him, humming or singing to him, watching for any sign of life, and trying to stave off reversals.

Although we felt Death lurking in the shadows of that first night, my mind held the door tightly against Death's press. I have no notes in my journal about that night, even though many years later the sense impressions seem as vivid as yesterday's activities. Shock stalled my speculative capacities. I did not, for example, wonder about the accident. I did not lament that Erik had left home that morning, though I tried repeatedly to picture him as he had been when he walked out the door. I had no concern for the car. Even telephone inquiries from other passengers' families barely registered in my consciousness. I was restlessly searching for some transcendent ground on which to stand my watch.

By early morning the institutional routines that govern hospital activity replaced the small, though significant, gestures of compassion we had experienced during our night-long vigil. The whooshing sounds of rising and falling elevators, the rattle of glass test tubes in metal baskets being whisked efficiently down the halls by rubber-soled medical technicians, and the clatter of breakfast carts greeted us as day broke. At dawn the hospital workers' treatment of us changed dramatically. No longer were we two loving parents in understandable shock; instead we were cast into the line of anxious visitors who waited, like supplicants, for the twice daily access to the sanctum that held the traumatically mangled bodies and brains of our loved ones. A nurse told us that we would now be restricted to the rigorously enforced rule of only two one-hour visits each day. In short, within eighteen hours after the accident that changed Erik's and our family's lives forever, we were forced to navigate in, and find some balance among, three dimensions: the inner space of anguish, the medical space of experts and fixed rules, and the external space of everyday life.

Our initiation into the liminal space of anguish on the one hand, and the technological-medical environment on the other, was not mediated by mentors like social workers or chaplains and certainly not by doctors. No one in a position of authority would talk to us. No one would help. Instead, we desperately picked up random pieces of information about hospital procedures, personality idiosyncrasies of doctors, various kinds and degrees of injuries, and the progression of treatments and interventions from a few communicative nurses and other families on similar vigils at the trauma unit gates.

As we entered the second day a trauma unit nurse, concerned for our well-being and medical efficiency, told us to go home and get some rest since we couldn't see Erik again until 11:00 A.M. When we reminded her that we lived over an hour away from the hospital, she suggested that we might be eligible, as out-of-town family of a critically injured patient, to stay in the Ronald McDonald House across the street behind the hospital. Since getting rest was far less important to us, whose vigorous, bright son now lay in stony silence, than it was to medical personnel, for whom this was simply another routine intake in the trauma unit, we put off investigating accommodations until later. We wanted to talk to a doctor.

But seeing a doctor was not easy. The physician who had performed Erik's surgery did not reappear during the night, though a trauma unit resident did stop by frequently to check on Erik, while one of us sat by his bed. He willingly answered informational questions but assiduously avoided any discussion about prognosis. By morning we had discovered that the trauma unit medical team of four doctors rotated shifts every twenty-four hours, each trying to stay abreast of every patient's condition. Interns, residents, and nurses also rotated on similar schedules. Though this organization may work well for the medical staff, it requires family members not only to comprehend a new medical language but also to interpret a wide range of communication styles and to fill in gaps that inevitably result when medical responsibility for patients is shared.

Finally, right before the eleven o'clock visiting hour, we found a doctor who reported that nothing had changed in Erik's condition since his arrival. We learned later from one of our relatives, a pediatrician who tried to get information from the hospital, that Erik's condition was described as critical for the entire first three weeks. The trauma unit physician reported that they had taken another CT scan during the morning and would have results later in the afternoon. In the meantime the staff would cool Erik's body to inhibit excessive swelling in the brain and watchfully monitor intracranial pressure. This was only the beginning of an endless chain of scans and X-rays and blood tests that hospital personnel would run on Erik. Clearly our son's physical care lay beyond our control. Even though outer appearances seemed to suggest that he was not registering our presence in any discernible way, Robert and I resolved not to abandon him. Questions poured from us. What was intracranial pressure? I made a layperson's guess that this referred to pressure on and around the brain caused by a severe assault to the head. Was there an acceptable pressure range? What were the consequences of pressure that exceeds that range? What factors would influence the rise of pressure?

During the first regular visiting hour we found ourselves in the strange company of the similarly distressed, a company that would expand and contract over the next three weeks and that we would come to experience as a wounded community. A mother and father called loudly and impatiently to their young adult daughter in a bed next to

Erik, imploring her to wake up. Within a few hours of Erik's arrival a girl just his age was admitted, having been thrown from a horse. For several nights one of the patients in the unit had police protection.

Looking for any clues that might help me negotiate through the unfamiliar world of trauma and among such a diverse group of waiting penitents, I instinctively became an unabashed eavesdropper. I listened to new words, asked for definitions, or wrote the terms in my journal to search for later; I overheard comments about kinds and locations of injuries; I learned about the Glasgow Coma Scale for measuring depth of coma and levels of responsiveness in three areas: motor response, eye-opening, and vocal response. Erik registered at the least responsive level. He showed no motor response, no eye-opening, and no vocal response, giving him a score of 3.[1] We began to talk to other parents and spouses as we waited together prior to visiting hours. We rapidly learned that most traumatic brain injuries occur to the young—most frequently to people between the ages of fifteen and twenty-five. Many injuries occur on motorcycles or in automobiles and involve guns or alcohol; secondary complications from delayed bleeding inside the brain, other injuries, seizures, repeated surgeries, or infections are common, and there is no predictability in the course of recovery from traumatic brain injury. As if these discoveries were not sufficient to depress us, most of the medical personnel were routinely pessimistic about favorable long-term outcomes, especially given the early ambiguity about the extent of damage to Erik's brain stem. While we desperately desired reassurance for our fear and grief, we instead moved more deeply into a terrain where violence, danger, and terror lurk and from which we had been largely insulated most of our lives.

After lunch on Monday, as I maintained our vigil outside the trauma unit, Robert made arrangements for us to stay in the Ronald McDonald House for what we naively hoped would be only a night or two. The urban setting mirrored the psychic state we were experiencing. Headquarters for the Campbell Soup industry, Camden was in visible decline. Some streets near the hospital looked like a war zone; poverty and crime held many city residents hostage. Guards and electronic monitoring systems protected hospital entrances, and we were advised not to walk across the street to the Ronald McDonald House after dark without a guard.

During this first twenty-four-hour, Memorial Day watch, Mike and his wife, Pat, returned with our daughter, a few overnight supplies, and a list of people they had called and others who had heard of Erik's injury and had called them. Even though we could not register the details of the calls reported to us, I felt increasingly, if precariously, upheld by a web of human connection quite distant from the hospital. At noon Richard came to see Erik and to offer freely his knowledge about head injury. In contrast to the trauma unit doctors, and perhaps to sustain his own hope, he was encouraged that Erik's condition had not worsened. "Severe injuries can result in responselessness," he counseled, "but the intricacies and mysteries of the brain make it impossible to predict anything for the next day, let alone weeks or months distant." He confirmed what we had already picked up in overheard conversations and doctors' responses: damaged parts of the human brain do not regenerate, but sometimes new connections can be made. Erik's was indeed a very serious injury but, our friend observed, his youth and physical fitness were in his favor. Although he said nothing as he lifted Erik's eyelids to look for any eye reactivity and as he pressed and pinched various places on his body, I interpreted his silence as his own uncertainty. His most reassuring words were that he would come again later that evening.

We had learned a few extremely sketchy details about the accident when we had arrived the previous day at Kessler Hospital. First among our concerns was how Erik had gotten from the adviser's car into the car of a young, inexperienced driver. This dismayed and angered us— we had given him specific instructions to ride with the adviser, and he had left the meeting house in the adviser's car. Apparently, as the group neared their destination, they had loaded another canoe onto the adviser's car. When the car dragged too close to the ground, one of the passengers was asked to move to the other vehicle for the two-mile trip to the river. Perhaps because of Erik's kindness or willingness to be co-operative, he was the one to move to the other car. As a result of that fateful decision, and despite the short distance, Erik's life now hung in the balance.

By our second evening in Camden we had received numerous calls in the trauma unit waiting area from family and friends wanting to know about Erik and expressing their concern. What could they do? Our parents, who were devastated by the news of what had happened to their first grandchild, wondered if they should come. We asked them not to but to keep hope alive for his survival and healing. We urged them to hold mental pictures of Erik strong and healthy in their minds and to gather around them some of their friends who could wait with them even at a distance of 700 miles. I knew at the time, and they confirmed it subsequently, that it was hard for them to remain helplessly at home. But we knew that we could not care for both their needs and Erik's in these critical circumstances.

At the close of the Monday evening visiting hour we finally looked at several scans of his brain with one of the trauma team doctors. With these visual images to examine, we were learning to decipher yet another language. How could I assimilate this smudgy two-dimensional image? Did that dark representation of a spherical mass of cells, presumably laced together with invisible neurons and synapses, belong to my son? I didn't know what the interior of an uninjured brain looked like, so how could I interpret the splotches that appeared under the lights as we viewed the scans? I felt overwhelmed by this new visual information, yet I tried to grasp, or infer, as much as I could. Despite the doctor's intention to inform us at least minimally about the brain's organization and function, these documents belonged to the initiated. Through them the doctor conveyed his authority and expertise as my own sense of powerlessness to aid my son increased hour by hour.

The scans showed diffuse, as opposed to localized or focal, bleeding in all parts of the brain, with special concentration in the frontal and temporal lobes. Indications about the extent and consequences of brain stem involvement were ambiguous. It was too early to predict the long-range implications of the injury. I desperately tried to grasp and hang on to the words the doctor was saying, but only later did I fully understand the physiological operations of the brain and its response to traumatic injury. Upon impact, Erik's brain had been jostled sharply from side to side inside the bony skull. Such wrenching movement produced bleeding from blood vessels throughout the brain. Blood had leaked into the surrounding tissue and was causing edema, which put additional pressure on the injury site and contributed to further swelling. Brain cells deprived of their blood supply die and do not regenerate, I heard the doctor explain. In addition, the dying tissue creates toxins that further exacerbate the swelling. Much depended on how the bleeding might be reabsorbed by the brain and whether swelling could be held at a minimum, thereby reducing further damage from intracranial pressure.

From asking several different nurses and residents during the first twenty-four hours I was beginning to understand that intracranial pressure occurs when the injured brain swells inside a fixed space—the skull—thereby causing a kind of compression chamber for the brain. The initial questions about direct damage to the brain stem at the time of the accident were now compounded by the problem of swelling, for edema can push the brain stem, which governs all the vital bodily functions, down into the spinal canal, producing a kind of herniation. To protect against such swelling Erik was kept on a cooling blanket, through which cooled water constantly circulated. It was clear that Erik was still very much in crisis. The doctor said developments during the coming week would provide better, important indicators of the true nature of his condition. None of the doctors was optimistic, although this particular one was, at least, kind.

We reported this discouraging news to Sonia and our friends, who were waiting both for some report from the doctors and for discussion about how to balance Sonia's need to complete the school year and ours to be close to Erik. If there were other options (and I imagine now that there were), we did not think of them, for Sonia thought she could, and wanted to, get back to school. Since 1981 and the founding of a small house church in Princeton, Pat and Mike Cox had become like surrogate parents or an aunt and uncle for our children. Their presence with us from the receipt of the fateful phone call onward provided us with essential strength and the courage simply to carry on. They had already said that they would provide a home for Sonia and transport her back and forth to school each day. Making these arrangements for the week ahead heightened our awareness that we would be staying in Camden for a while.

As we parted that evening Sonia sadly and gently asked, "What about my birthday party? Can I still have that?" With sharp poignancy her questions reminded me that she and Robert had been fixing up the basement for her party on Sunday when I arrived with the news of Erik's accident. Everything other than Erik's status had simply dropped from our minds, but the life force of our twelve-year-old pressed onward within her. Yes, we agreed that she should have the party, but we did not know how we would manage preparations that had barely begun. Exceedingly resourceful in every way—from hooking an old television to a videotape cassette player, to buying and preparing party food, to decorating a basement that was only partially cleaned, to helping our daughter feel as secure as possible in conditions that were inexplicably threatening—Pat and Mike quietly took over the at-home management of Sonia's overnight party, which was scheduled for the following Friday.

Reluctantly, with anxious hearts, we said good-bye again to Sonia, Pat, and Mike, and we left the hospital—the first time since we had entered it thirty hours earlier—and headed toward the Ronald McDonald House. The house itself was a lovely haven graciously hosted by a kind resident director and filled with caring guests. We asked the nurses to call us at the slightest change in Erik's condition at any hour, which they agreed to do. On the way out a rear exit we passed a vending machine snack shop and selected some soup and juice, a practice that would become habitual in the days and weeks to come.

Our sleep brought spaces of oblivion but little rest, for we were awakened repeatedly by the sirens of the ambulances bringing the injured and sick to the emergency room throughout the night. Each arrival startled us out of sleep to face the reality of a bad dream from which we could not escape. We were relieved when dawn broke and we could "reasonably" call for a report on Erik's condition. "No change," came the response. No worse. No better. Still critical. More waiting. By 8:30 we resumed our watch outside the trauma unit.

Although we didn't realize it at the time, our actions on the second morning in Camden would, over the coming weeks, take on the character of ritual. Upon rising we telephoned the unit, then showered, dressed, and ate breakfast in the hospital cafeteria. Well before 11:00 we were in the waiting area, usually sitting by ourselves unless a new patient had just been admitted. For both of us, being close by was important. We sat in silence, writing perhaps, praying or meditating. Frequently we received phone calls, and we would repeat the story another time or report "no change." Often during the first week I retreated to the small bathroom off the waiting area when the weight of my anxiety and grief became publicly unbearable; there I could hurl my anguish soundlessly at the walls.

On Tuesday morning Robert returned a call we had received from the police department. The officer was kind as he inquired about Erik, asked about insurance matters (New Jersey was a no-fault state), and then proceeded to explain that the driver of Erik's car had made a left-hand turn across two lanes of moving traffic. Apparently his view had been obstructed by a van that was waiting to make a left-hand turn from the opposite direction, or perhaps he thought he could get across the lane in which an oncoming vehicle was traveling. The car was hit broadside at the back door, right where Erik was sitting, and was propelled into a telephone pole on the opposite side. The car was so compressed that the Jaws of Life were required to extricate Erik. Questions about the speed at which the oncoming vehicle was traveling were ambiguously answered. Before the call ended, however, the police officer advised us to get a lawyer, a need that seemed inconceivable at the moment, given our focus on the immediate survival of our son.

This additional information about the circumstances of the accident troubled us deeply. The previous day the eighteen-year-old driver of the car in which Erik had been riding had come to the hospital with his father, and I had felt immediately torn. I was incredulous that Erik was the only one who had been severely injured in the accident. I also struggled with anger that somehow Erik chose or had been chosen to move to this young man's car. Then I felt compassion for what I imagined I would be feeling if I were in the driver's shoes. The father and son expressed their regret, and Robert and I hurried to tell them not to blame themselves. Now, after Robert's conversation with the police officer, we realized that Erik's driver, although inexperienced rather than reckless, bore significant responsibility for the crash. Anger sank more deeply into our hearts, sat beside our grief, and confounded the charity.

Later on Tuesday a trauma physician asked our permission to perform a tracheostomy on Erik—a procedure to open his trachea for air passage. We hesitated, for we knew the risks involved—possible direct damage to the vocal cords or later compromise from scar tissue. We deduced from his request that the medical team thought Erik was not on the verge of waking up. The doctor explained the comparable hazards of leaving the nasal tube in place, and so we gave our permission to perform the surgical procedure. Facing choices with equally undesirable outcomes would become commonplace over the next weeks and months.

Waiting to see Erik each day created profound anticipation, even excitement, for we kept believing that this time he would surely awaken. Although the excitement was mingled with dread, the feelings were similar to those that I had experienced immediately after giving birth, when I wanted to see and hold this unknown being who had come forth from my flesh. To quiet myself and to find inner resources for facing the unknown, I tried to meditate. Often it was impossible to still my active, pleading mind. Why? Why? What is the meaning of this? What had

Erik done to deserve this fate? I had come unwittingly to rely on reasonableness in life, and this event simultaneously exposed and subverted that illusion. During these attempts to meditate I wanted to visualize Erik as I had remembered him just two days before. I could not. I could recall topics of conversation or an article of clothing; I was able to remember his activities the day or two before the accident; but I could hold no unitary picture of our son in my mind's eye. It was as if my own memory cells had been damaged by his injuries.

Quickly the rituals of meditating and waiting to see Erik anchored our lives, which edged close to disintegration. When we were with Erik my anxiety abated because I had his physical presence with which to communicate. I was grateful when the medical staff would leave us alone with him so that we could speak freely with him. Yet these one-hour visits were also the only times we could easily seek information or ask for interpretation. We learned to read and interpret the monitors just as expectant parents listen for the heartbeat of their in utero child or view its image by means of ultrasound. We observed closely when doctors or nurses looked at his pupils to see if they responded to light and, by asking questions, learned crudely to detect their reactivity. But from Erik, no response.

During much of the time we spent with Erik we found ourselves relating to him as we did when he was first born. Now, however, he was somewhere far beyond our reach, and he gave us no clues about his needs. Nonetheless, we spoke to him gently, telling him each time we came who we were and that we loved him, reassuring him when we had to leave that we would be either just outside in the waiting area or across the street and only a phone call away. We routinely caressed his head and limbs. Amid the tubes and machines, I practiced the ancient technique of energy movement a few inches above his body. We told him about the good wishes of those who had called and suggested that he imagine these people all standing around his bed. From the depths of our spiritual reservoirs came unsolicited passages from the Psalms, childhood lullabies, lines from poems we had read when he was a child or that he had learned recently in school. Whenever we mentioned relatives or friends we would remind him of the person's relationship to him and describe a recent interaction or recall a special occasion with the individual. We sometimes included the monitors in our communication, reporting what we saw. Particularly when a sudden change registered, we asked him if he was frightened, in pain, or upset.

On one level, unconsciousness and the absence of speech may make such comments and questions seem ludicrous. Yet at another level we sensed we were engaged in a new form of communication that was directed largely by our instincts, our bodies, and the impression that we had to reach behind the veil of language and consciousness to seek our son. As our visiting time drew to a close we would usually hum quietly to him, pray a very simple prayer, and reassure him of our continuing nearness to him even when we were physically absent. Each day these meetings briefly grounded our lives.

Often in class discussions and in teaching writing I have counseled students to risk vulnerability by disclosing their thoughts and feelings, which could help them discover their own values and ideas and communicate them clearly. As our son hovered in these early days between life and death, I learned how wide the chasm is that separates vulnerability that is chosen from vulnerability that crashes upon us. The impact of what was happening to us dawned on us by degrees. Our first reactions of terror and disbelief registered physically in persistently knotted stomachs, grief lumps in the throat, and restless sleep. Our identification with our son produced vicarious pain and a continuous feeling of powerlessness to mitigate what we imagined he might be going through, even while unconscious. In an instant all the care and caution with which we had protected our children were rendered irrelevant, and we could do nothing to change that reality. This vulnerability promised no clarity, but threatened to reveal meaninglessness.

The accident disturbed the family nest for each of us as father, mother, or sister, or even grandparent, aunt, uncle, or cousin. When we spoke to our relatives and our friends on the telephone we heard, in their voice tones if not in their words, their troubled efforts to make some kind of sense of an event that seemed so incomprehensible and so unjust. I frequently wondered how Sonia was experiencing and processing this assault on the family system.

As we grasped for our psychic centers and the spiritual resources to carry us through this enforced vulnerability, we had to learn to read the signs, language, and ways of organizing medical knowledge. We had to construe meaning for medical information encoded in specialized jargon and cryptically hidden in case notes usually not available—or, if available, virtually undecipherable—to patients or their families. We had simultaneously to tolerate the depersonalization of our son and resist the routine that turned him into an object analyzed by medical professionals.

Those who cared for our son and kept records on him were in effect telling a story about him. Their protocols, the tone of their voices, their investigation and interpretation of the data about his condition acquired from the machines—indeed, the pervasive impersonality and instrumentality of most relationships in the trauma unit—dismayed us and reduced Erik to a body struggling for survival. In these circumstances I felt like a wandering soul cast into Limbo, the first circle of Dante's hell.

Each day Erik's and our vulnerability deepened and manifested itself in new ways. In retrospect I understand that as the gap widened between the hospital and the strawberries left in the kitchen and the work abandoned on our desks, we became engaged in a cosmic struggle not simply between good and evil, as we understood them, but more wrenchingly between love and perfection. This struggle appeared in various guises. Sometimes Robert and I experienced it together as a contest between our need to relinquish everything and our mutual desire to control outcomes. Often we found it expressed in our differing responses to the crisis. There was no doubt that we both loved deeply, but through our separate styles of coping with fear and grief, we sometimes grew impatient with each other. Robert's take-charge rationality and desire to fix whatever breaks down or falls apart clashed with my need to turn inward to process my feelings and to persist in calmly attempting to communicate with the spirit of our injured son. In the confusing throes of anger, fear, and heartbreak, each of us clung tenaciously to the hope that, through our love and will, perfection would kiss our son's brokenness and return him as we knew him.

During these first four days, the persistence of our hope for restoration to perfection illustrated both our naivete about traumatic brain injury and our denial of the severity of Erik's particular injury. We struggled mightily with the temptation to measure love's efficacy by images of perfection. Never before had we confronted anything our love could not protect, control, or improve. On this threatening threshold we waited.

Waiting in Crisis

The journey launched permitted no U-turns.
Each morning anxiety and grief
knocked on our bodies,
threatening to surpass
physical stamina and spiritual resources.
One step upon another
I repeated simply "I must go on."

As I awoke each day with hope, showered, and crossed the street that separated the few remaining routines of an ordinary life from the world of the medical establishment to wait for news of some change, I endured from moment to moment by acknowledging that I had to hang on. Those intense, confusing feelings found form in my journal, two and a half years later.

MEMORIAL DAY

James Agee described it first
in Rufus who lost his father

over a cliff—a bolt loosed
in the steering column—
that feeling of importance
bestowed through death
in the family.
Shamed and condemned by the universe,
Rufus-in-me tiptoed to
whoosh, blip, and purr;
Anger and Grief
played on my ribs,
blew out my heart,
cut circulation to
death-nipped extremities,
while on Memorial Day
I waited for you to know
whether to return or go.

For Sonia, the waiting to know whether her brother would "return or go" was both more distant and more emotionally intense than she was developmentally able to recognize or we attentive enough to fathom fully. While Robert and I hovered around Erik in the hospital, trying to maintain some slender connection with his physical form and spirit as we remembered it and to interpret the discourse of the medical professionals, Sonia returned to Princeton and the "real" world. Though she lived at Pat and Mike's home each evening and stayed in daily phone contact with us, the events of May 26 had separated her from the family as crisis moved the family circle away from home ground.

From that developmental and geographical distance she too tried to incorporate this encounter with the odious into a stable world. On May 7, twenty days before Erik's accident, Sonia had started to keep a diary—a red, clothbound book into which she intended to record her thoughts and feelings as she experimented with the power of language.

One day I saw a tree
and it said to me,
"do not flee," he said
"for thee
shall see
me."

        S.J. 6/19/84

Diary, Happy Mom's Day! Today was really super! I went to Meeting with Brian and our family and made gingerbread which was a success and after Meeting went to Lover's Lane Park for a picnic, and we bought some subs which were good. We looked at some trees and Mom found a bench that was strange and she started swinging her legs! She looked like a little girl. We all played Frisbee and then came home. I started feeling sick and then House Church came and I felt better soon. I have a track meet tomorrow, so I need to go to sleep.

Diary, Today was a normal day except I'm really mad and sick of Kim. She always thinks that she's the best and she's always right. But I'm not going to let her silly ideas and distractions bother me. Right now I'm just sticking to my feelings and no one else's. . . .

Diary, Wow! Guess what? There is a HUGE thunderstorm going on outside and there was a huge pop and the lights dimmed. It's really exciting. It's pouring. Well, today we finished the CATs and they were pretty fun. Believe it or not! OOH! That was a loud one. Cathy is sticking with Melvyn and they are very fine. I'm sort of unhappy because I found out that G.M. started going out with somebody just today . . . an 8th grader. Oh, well, you lose some and you win some. I'm going back to watching the thunderstorm. P.S. I'm making plans for my birthday.

May 25, 1985. Diary, Mom and I woke up around 7:30 this morning and went to pick 6 quarts of strawberries. We then came home and had pancakes, bacon and strawberries for breakfast. Yummy! Then we planted some geraniums out front and I went to my viola lesson and string quartet picnic and even Junko was there. She told us about when she was young and she played the violin. She never really thought about having a choice to play . . . she just did. Good night.

 As a mother looking back on my young daughter's experiences in 1985 and still further back to my own feelings and growing awareness at twelve years of age, I can only ask of Sonia and my long-ago self, "What were you going through?" That question and her innocent diary provide a continuo over which the hours and weeks that would lengthen into months of waiting for her brother would be played out.

In my recollections of my twelve-year-old psyche, emotions seemed to lead my life. Any instant anger, sadness, exhilaration, or fear could arise and shift my balance as I teetered between childhood and incipient maturity. Unlike the volatility characteristic of many emotions, however, traumatic shock settles in the belly and puts paralyzing pressure on the brain. Sitting in the back seat close together on the way to the hospital, for example, Sonia and I were held together in the clutches of fear. Noiselessly it took up residence with shock, chasing questions endlessly around my mind. Sonia, in contrast, sat in wordless incredulity, looking out without seeing the towns or freshly seeded fields we passed, hearing yet simultaneously blocking out the anxious words of her father in the front seat as fear carried her toward an abyss of the unknown. As she waited that first afternoon and evening in the emergency room of one hospital and then in the surgical unit corridor and the trauma unit waiting area of a second, watching strangers come and go around her, seeing us disappear behind large doors or be ushered into small rooms and then reappear to report on what we'd been told or to consult with Pat and Mike, she seemed, to us and perhaps herself, to become invisible in the large arms of fear.

Sonia was from an early age a good reader both of word texts and of people. Her own initial shock, plus her ability to intuit the clues about the severity of her brother's condition from the faces and voices of those around her combined with our preoccupation and barely conscious effort not to let ourselves and her be totally overwhelmed by fear, reduced our communication the first day and night to cryptic exchanges. When we returned to her in the emergency room waiting area after our first sight of Erik and our first conversation with the attending physician, she asked, "Is he going to be all right?"

What did it mean in her young mind for him *not* to be all right? Was she imagining his not being at all? As his mother who had labored to bring him into being, I could, but could *she*, for whom he was as much a part of her being perhaps as her own body and breath?

After the trauma surgeon who performed emergency surgery at the Camden hospital reported that he had been able to repair the spleen and that the heart, lungs, and liver seemed not to have been compromised she again said, "That's good news, isn't it? Does that mean he'll be all right?"

At the end of that first day she wrote in her diary:

I am so scared. . . . The day started out well. Dad and I were cleaning and decorating the basement for my party, and then Mom and Pat and Mike came in and said Erik had been in an accident . . . Mom and Dad are a wreck. Dad was crying and Mom just looked horror stricken . . . I'm just praying that Erik will get better because I'd miss him a lot if he didn't. . . . P.S. Pray for Erik.

As we struggled on Memorial Day to focus our scattered attention on how Sonia could return to school without us, for what we thought would only be the next few days, she outwardly conveyed assurance, even confidence, that she would be all right staying with Pat and Mike. The three of them left the hospital with a key to stop at our house to pack a few clothes and pick up Sonia's books.

Thinking about Sonia after she left with Pat and Mike, I imagined what she had to face in going home and wrote in my journal:

The house must feel eerie to her, almost as if someone has died. All the stuff we dropped and left behind . . . only yesterday? . . . will be in the same place. A hammer by the basement door. The strawberries probably still in the re-frigerator waiting—to be cleaned, to be eaten, to be frozen? It will be dark when they get home, and she'll have to go upstairs alone. How she used to be afraid to go up alone at night when she was little! I wonder if she'll look in

*Erik's room, the very lived-in (she'll call it messy) quality just the way he left
it. Does he know he's been in an accident? Did he know it was happening?
Where is he now? These are maybe my questions, not Sonia's. She'll wonder
what to take to Pat and Mike's. How much for how long? She'll wonder about
her party. Oh, to be with her there and also here!*

From her developing inner world Sonia negotiated between a junior
high school environment that stayed frustratingly the same as she had
come to know it, and a medical world of crisis with which she had only
phone contact and visits to her parents. The typical concerns of seventh-
grade girls—Are my clothes as good as everyone else's? How should I
style my hair? Who likes whom? Who is angry with whom?—plus academic pressures had been troubling Sonia before the accident. When she
returned to school after the Memorial Day holiday and walked into the
commons of her large suburban junior-senior high school, though everything remained the same in outer form, inwardly nothing was the same.
Alone later she wrote in her diary:

*Diary, Erik is staying the same and I'm getting a little lonely for everyone.
Everyone at school was concerned and they were sympathetic and that made
me feel good. I have a science test tomorrow and Mike helped me study again.
The math test wasn't too hard . . . Tomorrow Dad is going to come home for
a day from the hospital to spend it with me. Mary's birthday party is on Friday and Dad and I or Pat and I are going to get her a gift tomorrow maybe . . .
Keep praying.*

*Diary, Erik is basically the same and Dad came from the hospital today to see
me. He told me that after the car Erik was riding in got hit it went off the
road and hit a telephone pole. Erik's brain got injured in almost the worst
place possible—the stem which controls most of the functions of his body. I
got a 100% on my math test. Yeah! Dad and I got Mary earrings and records.
Dad says E.C. doesn't even respond to pain.*

*Diary, Mom and Dad called tonight. I wish they'd said Erik had woken up.
Instead they said no change. They told me about buying tennis shoes for Erik.*

I don't get it, but it's supposed to help. Seems funny to think of wearing shoes in bed.

Toward the end of the first week a trauma unit nurse and a resident physician advised that we bring some socks and a pair of high-top tennis shoes for Erik. I had vaguely noticed that other patients in the unit were wearing tennis shoes, indeed a bizarre sight, but had not inquired why. Now we learned that putting the shoes on and taking them off at two-hour intervals helped to prevent contractures of the feet and ankles that inevitably threaten patients who are immobile for prolonged periods of time. Erik did not own a pair of high-tops. Because we were not in our hometown and because neither Robert nor I wanted to venture into the crass commercial world of K-Mart alone, we left the hospital on our mission to buy an ordinary pair of shoes.

The four lanes of rapidly moving vehicles, the congestion of the parking lot, and the general oblivion in which customers and merchants carried on an endless string of transactions made us cling close together as we wound our way silently to the athletic shoes. There we faced a ridiculous choice of style—canvas or nylon or leather. Which would be best? The thought of which would withstand wear, one common criterion we had characteristically applied for such purchases in the past, brought a brief moment of laughter to lighten the pathos of this trip to the store. We bought shoes and socks that we considered durable as a testament, I suppose, to our hope that one day Erik might again wear them to shoot baskets on the driveway of our house. Inundated by powerlessness to assist our son, we attached near sacramental significance to selecting a pair of shoes.

Diary, no change. Tonight Mom and Dad said the doctor put a bolt in Erik's head. Gruesome. Where? Did they drill a hole? It freaks me out to think about this. They said this would help to measure pressure in the brain from swelling. Can Erik feel this? I just wish he'd wake up. Will he remember any of this when he wakes up? P.S. Keep praying. P.P.S. I haven't seen Mom for a whole week.

I missed Sonia intensely and worried about her in and out of the long hours of waiting outside the trauma unit. I looked forward to hearing her voice each evening, and as I wrote to Erik in my journal I assumed that somehow she was always listening in.

I have not been able to find you in my mind's eye, Erik, as you were— doing karate kicks, stirring up brownies or chocolate chip pan cookies, or explaining your house design for architecture class—because I am so afraid. . . .

In the times I could directly express my love and strength to Erik through touch, to Sonia in words over the phone lines, or to both in silent meditation, the grip of fear loosened, even if only momentarily. Separated by distance, Sonia and I each went on writing.

Diary, I think this has been one of the hardest weeks in my whole life. The stuff that my friends think is important is stupid. It makes me angry. I talk to Mom and Dad every night. I asked tonight about my party, and they said of course I'd still have it. But I don't know when we'll get ready for it. I really want it to be special. Dad gives me all the details from the day at the hospital. Mom does too, but she asks more about how I'm feeling and says to keep sending healing images to Erik. P.S. I wrote an essay a long time ago on Ali and me, and I got one of the highest grades possible . . . One week till my birthday!

Toward the end of the first week, arriving for our typical midday visit, we discovered a boltlike fixture sticking two to three inches out of Erik's skull at the hairline of his forehead. Though we were alarmed to observe that this device had been inserted into Erik's skull, the medical staff matter-of-factly assured us that the procedure was common when coma persists. The bolt registered the degree of intracranial pressure produced by swelling of the brain. By keeping watch on the bolt, the medical staff could intervene with medication or cool compresses to the head, raise the ventilator settings, or consider more drastic responses if the pressure rose outside a "safe" limit.

As Sonia went back and forth to school each day that Erik's coma persisted, Robert and I spent long periods of time together in silence, each trying to map the terrain of medical crisis with our individual resources. Robert kept a detailed record of every medical conversation and a list of

questions that arose each time we saw Erik. In a parent's version of doctors' case notes, Robert summarized his observations and recorded messages from the machines and devices like the bolt and from the medical
experts. Attentive to details and needful of control, he was the chief nav-
igator on these rough seas, scrutinizing the outward conditions sharply.
By contrast, my journal of the first ten days of crisis contained only spare
reports of Erik's daily condition but included a collage of poems, letters
to my son, and reflective efforts to make sense of the totally unsensible.

SUMMER MIDNIGHT

Is this crucifixion,
Mary? I now know as you knew,
pray for me—catholic in experience —
now in this hour of my grief.

TRAUMA UNIT

I long to scream,
leap, fear-maddened,
through the windows
(as the unknown one
from Cooper's fifth
tried last night)
instead I wait
politely
strangling terror
in my throat.

As I sought some firm inner ground on which to stand, Robert was rigorously challenging all outer orders as inadequate and unreliable and
questioning the architect of the universe who permitted the unjustified
suffering of innocents. Robert's willingness to express his anger and his
fear vociferously often angered me, for I experienced it as unproductive,
as a burden to my own similar but restrained emotions, and even as an
obstruction to the positive energy I believed we needed to channel to Erik.

Dad and Mom are totally absorbed in Erik. My needs or fears seem pretty small compared to him. They see everything through the eyes of the accident. I guess I'm glad that I have school to think about sometimes. I just want everything to be OK.

On the first of June, six days after the accident, as I picked up my spoon and put it to my mouth at breakfast—a movement I had performed without a moment's reflection for forty years—I marveled at the awesome complexity of the brain and human nervous system. Immediately from that thought I found my attention drawn to the cars being driven on the street two stories below the cafeteria windows. Behind each moving vehicle sat an adequately functioning human brain that prevented the vehicles from becoming a tangled mass. Unbidden observations like these occurred frequently; my awareness of every typical function of human interaction was acutely heightened. To me the world seemed charged with energy and power that sometimes sustained me and other times devastated me. Our lives felt like the wheels of an overturned vehicle that spin in the air after it has come to a crashing halt. All around us the intricate network of human traffic and discourse continued as we waited and hoped for our family vehicle to touch firm ground again.

After I took my viola lesson this morning Pat and Mike and I went to Camden. My recital is coming soon. Ms. Montanye says that I play very maturely. Unfortunately, Erik has had a setback. There was some more bleeding in the brain. . . . When we first saw Mom and Dad I knew something was really wrong. Mom was telling Dad what went on in the Trauma Unit after the nurses kicked him out. I don't understand it all, but something showed that Erik's brain pressure was rising, and it was in the danger zone. Dad wanted the nurses to call the doctor but they didn't want to until they tried dealing with the problem themselves. I was scared, but Mom said the pressure had come back down and they had called a doctor. Everything feels like it's falling apart, and Erik seems farther away somehow.

On June 1, when we entered for our noon visit, we discovered that because Erik had not shown signs of deterioration the nurses were trying to decrease his dependence on the ventilator. While we were with him, however, his intracranial pressure began to rise past what was safe. His blood pressure also began to rise, which set off an alarm that brought his attending nurse to his bedside. At first she calmly began what appeared to us to be an inappropriately slow investigation of the circumstances. As her minor adjustments produced no results in the monitors, we both began to panic, and Robert asked if a physician shouldn't be called, an inquiry that certainly could be regarded as a challenge to the nurse's competence or judgment. Caught between my desire not to distract the nurse from doing her job carefully and my own mounting fear, I tried to remain inwardly steady and to quiet Robert.

During the short time that Erik had been in the trauma unit we had become familiar with two procedures essential for the respiration of comatose patients: suctioning and bagging. The first procedure extracts excess mucous from the trachea and bronchial passages that a prone, motionless patient cannot remove; the second provides additional air, generated by a bellowslike device, for the patient's respiration when the ventilator is being adjusted. Erik's nurse began to "bag" Erik by hand, causing the pressure to drop slightly. But the pressure did not fall back into the normal range, and whenever the nurse paused the indicator of intracranial pressure would rise again. When Robert insisted that the nurse call a doctor, he was firmly asked to leave the unit. Since no one had spoken directly to me, I stayed, admonished by Robert as he departed to watch over these events closely. Despite the efforts of the medical staff to appear quite cool, this was clearly a turn for the worse, and no one gave us any suggestion as to what might be going on. When the nurse returned Erik to the respirator at the original settings, the crisis seemed to subside. Then the visiting hour ended, and I too had to leave without any knowledge of what was occurring. The doctor arrived just as I was leaving, and I told him he could find us in the waiting area.

A short while later the physician reported cryptically that he did not know what had caused the change. Did he really have no idea what had happened, or was he protecting his medical colleagues? The refusal to speculate without documentation, especially to parents, characterizes much medical discourse. He did venture that perhaps there had been more internal bleeding, though he thought that unlikely. He said he had ordered a CT scan, which might give some idea of what had transpired. By now we knew that additional swelling or bleeding portended further brain damage and made the prospects for recovery more bleak. Robert and I interpreted this change as ominous, and we called our families. We waited between the morning and evening visiting times without further reports, and Sonia and Pat and Mike decided to remain overnight with us. None of us said out loud that we feared Erik might die from this mysterious setback, but we knew that we needed to be together.

Dad and Mom wouldn't leave the waiting area all afternoon in case a doctor came by. I read a little, and then Pat and I walked around outside and looked in the gift shop. They asked me again if I wanted to go in to see Erik. I don't know. They don't press me to, so it's easier not to. I don't know what to expect, and I like to think of him as he was. But that is getting harder. He seems to be getting smaller.

We decided to stay overnight. After visiting hour tonight we ordered pizza at the Ronald McDonald House and talked about my party. Pat and Mike are great. Mike's going to fix up that big old TV Erik and Dad found junked so we can watch a movie in the basement. Pat will get the food, and they'll help me decorate. Mom and Dad promised that at least one of them would be there for sure. I know this is a small deal compared to Erik but it's important to me. It would be great if Erik could be better by my birthday, but I don't know if that's possible. I can't wait till I get to go home and things go back to normal. So must keep hoping and praying that Erik will get better. I love him. S.J.

In the evening, just prior to the visiting hour, we saw the neurosurgeon leave the trauma unit. When his eyes caught us in our usual spot, he stopped long enough to say that the scan had revealed additional spots of bleeding, but that it did not seem to be fresh bleeding. He thought it was a further effect of the initial injury showing up. Characteristically, he was not optimistic, stating that this puzzling development concerned him for the long-term prognosis. He said that the next twelve to twenty-four hours would be critical. We would have to wait to see if Erik could remain stable. The situation had been grim before this ventilator episode; now Erik's condition was more precarious.

Following the noonday incident, our confidence in the nurse who had been attending Erik at the time diminished, compounding our general anxiety with mistrust. She had finished her shift before we arrived for the evening, but it was apparent that everyone seemed more on alert than usual that night. Erik had stabilized after he had been returned to the ventilator, but he seemed very quiet and perhaps in a slightly deeper coma. No one spoke much to us, adding to our apprehension. Our attention on Erik during the evening hour was acutely focused; we held on to him in our hearts and tried to reach out to him wherever he was in deeper silence.

Today is Sunday, June 1. The sky is blue, blue, blue, and the birds are singing. One week since all this happened. It seems a lot longer. Mom and Dad and Mike went across the street to the hospital right after breakfast. No bad news about Erik during the night. That's good. Pat and I went to shop for some party decorations.

Soon after we had settled ourselves to wait for the two hours before visitation, Richard, along with the stepmother of the driver of the car in which Erik had been injured, arrived unexpectedly. We told them what had transpired, and then we all grew quiet as we waited together. All of us were familiar with silent meetings for worship in the tradition of the Society of Friends, so I was grateful that no one felt compelled to speak. Gradually I sensed the silence deepen and my own anxiety abate. In a fleeting inward observation I realized that we were experiencing what Friends call a gathered or centered meeting right here in the hospital alcove. As I allowed the silence to wash over me and seep into the aching folds of my heart, suddenly a very clear image of Erik in our family room gracefully practicing sharp karate kicks appeared. It was the first time in the week since the accident that such a complete inner picture had been possible. In that moment, paradoxically, I also felt able to relinquish him. If he left us, as I had been fearing throughout the long hours of the night, this image of my son as I had last known him would sustain me for whatever we had to endure. Perplexing as it sounds, even many years later, I knew on that Sunday morning, as Julian of Norwich proclaimed in the fourteenth century, that all would be well no matter what the outcome.

When we entered the trauma unit for our visit my extreme anxiety had been mitigated by the fresh image of Erik whole. Richard accompanied us and examined Erik's eyes with the attending nurse. His eyes were reactive, though not equally so, and his opinion was that Erik was not clinically worse than the last time he had seen him.

At the time of the ventilator crisis and since, our minds insistently sought explanations, either those given to us by professionals or ones that made sense to us as parents. During the instability itself we had wondered if the physical stress of breathing a few breaths per minute on his own put additional pressure on the brain stem, thus causing the rise in intracranial pressure. Perceiving how finely connected and dependent we are on cues that we receive from one another, I considered the possibility that our presence at Erik's side when his body was already under the stress of trying to resume its own breathing had diverted his "attention" or added some emotional pressure that triggered a rise of the intracranial pressure.

Many days later, upon hearing about the ventilator episode, one Quaker friend interpreted the continuing critical nature of Erik's condition as his spirit's wrestling with whether to stay in life or to depart. Convinced that in times of severe crisis the soul needs a space of rest and a kind of sorting out, or discernment, she advised us to wait patiently. Her interpretation made some sense to me on the spiritual and certainly symbolic level. Her confidence, however, that the boundary between life in the familiar physical forms through which we know it best and life in some much wider, cosmic-spiritual sense is permeable and that Erik's soul would make the right decision far surpassed mine at that time. Nonetheless, my capacity to wait with hope was enlarged by her wisdom.

Dear diary, only three more days till my party. Erik is now stable, but that's with all the tranquilizers in him. The doctors are watching him closely and now we have to wait and pray some more. Like I say, you can't have happiness without feeling pain. You can't have progress without feeling setbacks. It's not knowing what's going to happen that is scary. Could he die? What if he never wakes up? Lots of people call here at Pat and Mike's all day and all evening to find out about Erik. Some from really far away. Dawn and Mark are coming to our house Wednesday to help clean up the house for my party. Whoopee! It doesn't feel like my birthday. I wish I could have all my relatives come together for my thirteenth birthday, but I guess I can't.

Nearly every day, as we maintained our place in the trauma unit waiting area, we greeted friends who came by to see us or telephoned long-distance. Like the Friend who offered her interpretation of the ventilator incident, each one brought some gift from his or her storehouse of faith or wisdom, each speaking in his or her unique language of experience. One friend regularly read a Psalm to us and prayed for Erik and for us. Others recommended specialists of one kind or another or suggested books to read. Another friend with keen spiritual sensitivity encouraged me to look beyond Erik's physical absence by suggesting her own faith that his spirit was well and free. She explained that I could have conversations with his spirit, for she was already doing so herself.

Mom said that a friend of hers from twenty years ago had driven two and a half hours to see them at the hospital. Her own daughter the same age as Erik died last winter. I don't know why. And Mrs. Stoltzfus and Mr. Bing came too. Wow! I'm still keeping positive thoughts. I'm getting homesick. I wish things would be back to normal. I wonder if I'll get much for my birthday. Probably not. That's O.K., I guess. P.S. Keep praying.

One afternoon a woman about my age emerged from the elevator. She looked familiar, though she was walking with a cane. When she spoke my name with a question in her voice, I knew she was indeed Susan, whom I had not seen for at least twenty years. A vague recollection of having read in a church newsletter that her daughter, exactly Erik's age, had died several months earlier quickly crossed my mind. I did not know what the cause of death had been, and now here she stood before me, the mother obviously injured herself. Acquainted with grief and recovering from two broken legs sustained in an accident, Susan avoided the temptation to recount her own losses. She had driven two and a half hours to ask how she might help us.

With every such contact it became increasingly apparent that, despite how isolated we were from medical personnel and adequate information inside the hospital, we were not in this dark valley alone. Around the edges of this strange new world each friend spoke to us through language and experiences that were uniquely his or hers. Because my own integrated neural networks seemed severely disturbed by the trauma of brain injury to a beloved member of my family, I sought desperately to weave together some explanation or interpretation from these offerings that might uphold us in this confusion and disorientation. Gradually I discovered that I was taking a piece of yarn, as it were, from one friend's basket of suggestions and winding it with a piece from someone else's interpretation. Within the first week I had wound together strange medical terms, spiritual assurances, telephoned condolences, and personal visits from Erik's school adviser and the Princeton Day School headmaster, who told us who Erik had been to them and offered whatever help they could provide.

Daily, sometimes even hourly, new patterns in these gifts emerged as I connected and wove one into another or laid patches of others' advice and experiences next to each other. Not only were the friendships sustaining, but more important, I was winding and arranging the snippets of their experiences or reflections into a strong piece of fabric. As I regularly told Erik about the visits and telephone calls we received and described the outpouring of support and concern for him, I realized that I was creating a hammock made of human love and stories in which we were metaphorically holding him.

June 6, 1985. Diary, one day till teenage years! I'm not a child anymore; in one day! I'll miss that! I really will! Well, I've studied for my math test to-

morrow and I've decorated the basement at home. While I'm sleeping tonight, I'll turn 13! In a way I'm sort of unhappy because there really isn't anyone here to share my feelings with . . . Mom and Dad haven't called yet so I don't know what happened with Erik today. I pray all the time that he will get well. I wish things were the way they used to be. Hopefully, they soon will be! HAPPY 13, Sonia! I feel like no one is here to say good-bye to my childhood. I'm sad. Mom and Dad brought me into life, and they're not here to lead me out of my own childhood. I guess I'm really getting older!

Robert and I had discussed at length how to be present both for our daughter's important thirteenth birthday and with our critically injured son. We decided that I should go home and he would stay by Erik's side. Robert explained to Sonia his desire to be with her and his need also to remain with Erik, saying that he would make the same decision on her behalf if the situation were reversed. Though disappointed, she understood and later happily received his mid-party phone call.

When Friday dawned at the end of the second week, the day of Sonia's overnight party, I knew that I would have to mount a strong effort to leave the hospital and return to the house we had left in great dread when we learned of the accident. Late that night, back in our house for the first time since the accident, I wrote in my journal.

Erik, my son, I thought I could not stand to leave the hospital and to walk inside our house and see all the reminders of your wonderful, active, creative being. A note from Joy helped me to be aware of your spiritual presence, which in turn eased the reality of your physical absence. Oh, the irony, the agony — to be physically present but to feel so spiritually bereft. . . .

Pat and Mike had arranged for all the party food, had hooked up the salvaged television and the VCR in the basement, and had finished the decorations Sonia and Robert had been working on when we received news of the accident. I was required simply to be present and celebrate this important passage from childhood into adolescence with Sonia and her friends. I arranged to arrive at the house an hour before Sonia would get home from school so that I could enter the space and experience whatever emotions might arise in privacy. When I got out of the car I headed first to the backyard and the solace of the grove of trees behind the house. This outdoor space of lawn surrounded by tall trees had first attracted me to the property nine years earlier.

The backyard was quiet. The June sun and breeze played together on this my daughter's thirteenth birthday, pulling my memory back to our early autumn lunches on the swings when four-year-old Sonia returned from nursery school. Here we hauled in topsoil to build a raised garden which produced lettuce, green beans, and tomatoes along with pink petunias or bronze and yellow marigolds. Here we'd built snow people, played Frisbee and catch, and romped carefreely with Happy. Happy's dog pen is empty now; he's in a kennel. The barely planted garden is a bit more weedy. Nature never stops.

Looking toward the trees I saw the grand tree house, towering about twelve feet off the ground, that Erik and his friends had built the previous summer. Instantly I was overcome with pain and sadness, but in the midst of my tears I remembered the words of my friend who said that I could communicate with Erik's spirit. That thought reoriented my sense of loss. By calling up mental pictures of the ways Erik and his friends had scavenged for lumber from nearby building sites, salvaged old nails from the same sites or their dad's workshops, carried discarded carpet remnants from their homes to put the glorious finishing touches on a structure of which the youthful builders were all proud, I regained the boy I loved as I had known him. Even in absence, in these surroundings and through memory, he became gracefully present.

Without doubt, the two most difficult features of the birthday party were being fully present to Sonia's excitement and greeting her friends and their parents, who either did not know what to say or completely ignored the whole subject of Erik's injury. Struggling still with my own shock and denial, I again realized in this brief return to typical human interaction that I resided now on a threshold between two worlds—the medical world and the one I called my everyday world—without adequate means of communication for easy conversation in either one. If this was true for me, who still had consciousness and speech, how much more was this true for our comatose son? In the hospital I was regarded as invisible or of no consequence in the discourse of medical experts; in the world of everyday activities—where fathers and mothers go to work, kids go to school and soccer practice, and we are urged to buy and sell our souls into numbness—coma and brain injury did not fit. Pressing insistently and barely hidden underneath my sense of hovering between worlds lay our daughter's desire for her parents to accompany her as she walked across the threshold from childhood to adolescence.

On my return to Princeton for this twelve-hour stay I began to experience more acutely the difference between the medical case notes constructed by doctors and the biographical narrative we had lived with our son. The medical professionals were developing a story as well, though a more limited one, for they were concerned with investigating and ordering only a select set of intense events from the larger story of Erik's life. Though a medical plot usually depends on the presentations of the patient, from which the doctor selects the most salient or germane details for the plot, Erik was unable to contribute anything. Even the contributions we as parents might have made to placing the accident in a larger story were not sought by the medical professionals or social workers or chaplains. The plot of Erik's medical narrative was being recorded in case notes, which were beyond our reach. Constructed from interpretations of blood tests and x-rays and descriptions of surgical procedures, it was taking shape in the logs and charts, in doctors' rounds, and in staff discussions. The medical narrative emphasized the present, disregarded the past, and held any future in abeyance. It also protected itself, sometimes at the expense of us and Erik. By contrast, we intuitively continued to story Erik's life in the face of his silence, linking him to his past through the dread-filled present, and pressing in faith toward a future regardless of its uncertainties.

Diary, my party was great. Mom went back to Camden this noon. Tomorrow Aunt Sharon is coming. Mike will meet her at the airport and then she'll come to my recital. I am glad she's coming. Maybe she'll help Mom and Dad relax a little. I hope my piece goes O.K. I wish Mom and Dad could be there. They said I should play it for Erik.

As I returned to the hospital on Saturday afternoon, Sonia and Pat and Mike remained in Princeton to meet my sister, Sharon. She was flying in on Sunday from Minneapolis to help us keep our vigil with Erik and to attend Sonia's string recital. Sonia told me as I left that I should tell Erik that she would play her viola solo—the third movement of a Vivaldi concerto—for him. When Pat, Mike, and Sonia brought Sharon to the hospital following the recital, all agreed that Sonia's performance had seemed inspired.

Sharon was in the midst of a doctoral program in counseling psychology. Although the summer months afforded her a somewhat more flexible schedule, we knew that, because she was finishing her course work and looking ahead to comprehensive examinations, her schedule was still full. At first we resisted her offer to come, but I took solace and strength from her presence, which gave us a little space to rest since we knew that she would be an advocate on Erik's behalf whenever we were absent. Her sensitivity and acute ability to listen provided us with nurturing attention that is generally unavailable in the world of medical discourse.

With Sharon's arrival at the Ronald McDonald House at the beginning of the third week, we had settled in, albeit restlessly and anxiously, to a routine. We were becoming part of a community of parents who live on the margins of the medical world while caring for their children in crisis. Some of these parents came regularly to the hospital to monitor their children's diseases like leukemia or to wait with them as they received treatments. Some followed developments in severe disabilities present from birth. The great racial, economic, and educational differences in this marginal human community were leveled by our mutual needs. What I find most impressive in retrospect is how generally trusting of life these people seemed, despite circumstances that neither they nor their children deserved or sometimes could even understand. In our anguish and fear, Robert and I sometimes privately wondered how they could laugh or joke or watch television. Though all of us focused on our particular reason for living temporarily in this community, we inquired about the condition of one another's children as we passed in hallways, the laundry room, or the kitchen, each evening or at odd moments during the day.

From the second week onward I had begun regularly to record my "conversations" with Erik in my journal. As I was writing one such conversation outside the Ronald McDonald House in the warm mid-June sun I was called to the telephone. The neurosurgeon informed me that the most recent CT scan of the brain had revealed that Erik's left ventricle was shifting significantly to one side, a condition caused, he speculated, by a fluid buildup in the cranial cavity. He had already reserved the operating room for the following morning and advised prompt surgery to relieve this pressure, for he thought this condition might be contributing to the continuing depth of Erik's coma.

Diary, Well, the week of finals finally began. Science wasn't too hard and I've math tomorrow and I already studied all thirteen chapters. More bad news about Erik. Dad and Mom called tonight to tell me that the brain doctor thinks that there is pressure on the brain from fluid around the brain. He will do surgery tomorrow morning. I hope this helps. P.S. Keep praying.

We once again faced the need to relinquish our son to the medical professionals who were mediating between his life and us. We asked questions about the necessity of the procedure, the risks, and the consequences of not performing the surgery. Dependent on and grateful for the technological and medical expertise that we hoped would aid our son, we nonetheless met this new development anxiously. We consulted with our medical friend in Princeton by telephone, asking if the proposed procedure made sense. During the evening visit we calmly spoke to Erik about the condition the neurosurgeon had described to us. As we gently caressed his body and hummed childhood songs to him, we attempted to reassure him and prepare him for the surgery the next morning.

The nightly walk from the hospital across the street to the Ronald McDonald House represented the enforced separation from our son that we reluctantly endured. On this night before surgery we clung to each other more tightly as we released Erik to the skill of the doctor and the care of God, whom we sometimes felt like blaming even as we offered unbidden petitions to Him or Her and who, we were in fleeting moments beginning to believe, suffered with us. The uncertainties and ambiguities that engulfed us this particular evening reminded me of pregnancy, for now, as when I carried my unborn child in my womb, I did not know who the child would be or if he or she would arrive healthy. I felt now as if we were extending a second umbilical cord, this one a metaphorical one, as we waited for Erik's second arrival.

The following morning, as Robert, Sharon, and I waited in the surgical waiting room, we were joined not only in spirit by family and friends at a distance who knew Erik was having surgery but also by several people from the Friends Meeting who came and waited in silence with us. When the doctor emerged to report about the procedure he asked, "Are you still meditating?" The simplicity of that question and the respect with which I think it was posed allowed the medical narrative and Erik's story to touch briefly. In a fleeting moment of acknowledgment, we as parents mediated between Erik as a case report, constructed by remote multiple narrators, and Erik as the fifteen-year-old son of two anguished parents hoping for the restoration of their child. The neurosurgeon immediately returned to his customary mode of detached discourse. He confirmed that it had been a wise decision to do surgery because as soon as he drilled the hole in the skull, a spurt of fluid shot out, suggesting that there indeed was a buildup of internal pressure on the ventricles. Soon we were able to see Erik. We learned that he had gone through the surgery on a low ventilator setting and that his heart rate and blood pressure remained normal. The most noticeable difference we observed was that his eyelids were fluttering. We were overjoyed and wanted to dance through the hospital corridors. We imagined Erik watching us and laughing because we knew so little how to rejoice, not only in this moment but in many of life's moments.

Diary, the math final went pretty well and it wasn't too hard. Erik's surgery went well, Mom said. As soon as the doctor finished "drilling" the hole,

Mom said that the doctor said the fluid just shot out, so it probably was putting pressure on the brain and it was good to let it out. Mom also said they didn't need to give any "extra" breaths of air to E.C. during the surgery, which means that he mainly went through the surgery on his own strength. He is now on three breaths per minute from the respirator. Well, that's good news.

By the end of the third week Erik's eyes were opening more of the time, and he had gradually been removed from the ventilator and was breathing completely on his own. The blood gases were good, and the gastric feeding tube, which fed him directly into the stomach, was exchanged for one that ran from his nose into the stomach. We were overjoyed by the progress as we left him for the night. Instead of getting our standard evening fare of canned Campbell's soup from the snack shop, we decided to order a pizza and to look forward to the time when Erik could eat with us again.

Diary, I thought the social studies final was easy. A LOT OF NEWS ON ERIK. *I went down to the hospital with Pat today since I had only a half day. Mom, Dad, and Sharon greeted us and told us that this afternoon Erik opened one of his eyes and kept it open a little while. He then moved his hand down his leg, it seems because he was urinating and some of it wasn't going in the tube . . . Mom and Dad say that I should send a tape of me talking to Erik to the hospital. I'm going to tell him that he's got to wake up or I'll just figure he's chicken and doesn't want to beat me at "Around the World."*

Our guarded joy slid into the valley of fear two days later when Erik's left arm twitched involuntarily and unnaturally while we were visiting. As with so many symptoms that accompany brain injury and about which we learned after they had manifested themselves physically in Erik, I did not know what the brief spasm might mean. It was unnatural, unexpected, and alarming. The nurse attending him observed it closely, examined his eyes, and speculated that he had had a seizure. Once again we received yet more information about the consequences of brain injury. Seizures are quite common, we learned, and people who have sustained head injuries may need to remain on anti-seizure medications for the rest of their lives. By our next visit Erik was receiving Dilantin;

we knew about this medication and its negative side effects, particularly on the liver with prolonged use, from my mother's use of it to control a severe trigeminal neuralgia. Naturally we wanted to avoid seizures for Erik, but we also wished to protect him from weakening other still healthy organs in his body. Within the next forty-eight hours Erik began to break out with a rash, which the doctors immediately described as a reaction to Dilantin, so he was given Phenobarbital as an alternative drug. Fortunately, the medication controlled Erik's seizure activity, though we could never be sure if or when an episode might occur again. Throughout this brief spate of seizures I was perplexed by the optimism and encouragement that the medical professionals expressed when they could prescribe a medication or a technological intervention for some discrete need compared to their overall pessimistic attitude when we wanted to talk about Erik as a whole being, as our son.

The ambiguities of Erik's condition and the contradictions we experienced between our concern for him as a son and the medical care he was receiving threatened daily to defeat us. As we picked up new terminologies, tried to decipher rapidly spoken medicalese that we weren't always sure described our son, and resisted the temptation to interpret the doctors' or nurses' facial expressions or their silences, Erik was aided by medical protocols developed in warfare. A. R. Luria's investigations of brain-injured soldiers during World War II had been augmented dramatically by technological innovations developed on the combat fields of Vietnam.

Amidst the aggressive, often confusing technical-medical treatments, Erik and we also profited from a conversation that had been carried on for several weeks without our knowledge. We had not had the presence of mind to contact our hometown pediatrician about Erik's injury, but our physician's daughter, who was a classmate of Erik's, had told her father about the accident, and he had initiated regular contact with the trauma unit physicians regarding Erik's condition. Despite our lack of knowledge of this, our pediatrician performed a tremendous service to Erik and to us, for his interest provided another context of care and accountability. Concern for a patient registered by another physician encourages attending physicians to exercise their skills as fully as possible on the patient's behalf. When we learned from one of the attending trauma unit physicians that our doctor had been calling and had invited us to call him, we made contact immediately. He urged us to get a second opinion about Erik's condition from a pediatric neurosurgeon at the University of Pennsylvania hospitals, just across the river from Camden. In this important initiative by our pediatrician the personal and medical worlds intersected again.

Diary, the seventh grade trip to Great Adventure was great! I went on so many rides—all the "dizzy" ones. Mom and Dad called (really because they were checking to see if I was all right) and told me that Erik is about the same . . . I go down to the hospital tomorrow. I may go in to the trauma unit. I don't know, it's a little scary. Keep hoping.

On Saturday morning at the end of the third week, when we arrived as usual to wait for the noon visiting hour, we were greeted by two nurses leaving the trauma unit. They informed us that Erik was to be moved to the seventh floor and that arrangements were under way for the transfer. Once again we had not been informed by medical personnel or prepared for this significant transition. From one point of view such a move seemed precipitous, and we speculated together that trauma unit space must be needed for more critically injured people. When we asked the nurses whether they thought Erik was ready for such a move, they agreed that a few more days in the unit probably would have been desirable, but they felt he was stable enough to make it outside the unit. Upon entering the trauma unit we discovered that the move had already begun, and we had no choice but to join the procession of Erik in his bed and the accompanying equipment toward the seventh floor.

In the midst of our questions about why this transfer was taking place on the weekend, when hospitals generally operate with less than a full staff, Pat and Mike arrived with Sonia. Expecting to find us in the waiting area, they learned that we were moving with Erik to another floor. The path to the seventh floor was circuitous, but Pat, Mike, and Sonia followed it like detectives in a mystery novel seeking evidence of a body removed from the scene of a crime. Erik in his bed, with feeding pump, heart, blood pressure, and respiration monitors, nurses and his parents in tow, moved in and out of elevators and around corridors about ten or fifteen minutes ahead of Pat, Mike, and Sonia. Erik was first incorrectly sent to a wing that had not been prepared to receive him. As the surprised staff tried to make quick accommodation to take on this new patient, word came from somewhere that he was to go instead to a different wing on the same floor. All these maneuvers, confusingly directed from a disembodied source, unsettled us—we wanted to maintain the best possible care for our son. At the time of the move Erik had been continuing to open his eyes a little more regularly, though there was no engagement or apparent recognition in them. In the midst of the confusion over directions, we attempted to remain outwardly as calm as we could in order to reassure Erik, for his eyes, when they opened, seemed to register fear.

Somewhere in the middle of a hallway between the wrong and right rooms, all of us in a state of disarray, Pat, Mike, and Sonia found our entourage. Without our knowledge Sonia had decided that she was ready that day to visit Erik in the trauma unit. Because of these change-of-location developments, we had no time to support her decision or prepare her for her first visit with her brother. When we met Sonia in the hallway, I gasped inwardly, for she was meeting her profoundly changed brother with no opportunity to process her personal emotions in private or with us. What amazed me then and continues to impress me was the way she quietly moved straight to the bedside and softly touched Erik's hand.

Diary, . . . Erik looks like I thought he would except he's pretty skinny. He keeps having diarrhea so he can't keep much nutrition in him . . . I've learned to be able to talk to him and hold his hand. I told him about my party and he kept his eyes open a crack.

The significance of that simple gesture of touch became transparent to me only twelve years later when Sonia and I were being interviewed in New Zealand about the effects of brain injury on a family. During the interview Sonia explained that as a twelve-year-old her identity was heavily linked to her older brother. Because she knew no part of life that had not included his presence leading her, when he was injured it was as if a part of her had been yanked from her by the roots. Reflecting years later on this first post-accident encounter with Erik, Sonia remarked that she was reaching out to give some small aid or comfort to someone who now was no longer the brother she had known; through touch she defined herself as separate, though also maimed, and assumed a role of "older" sibling.

After our jagged detour we arrived on the north side of the seventh floor, and Erik was moved into a room with another comatose patient. Though the staff here had been informed of Erik's arrival, they were not fully prepared; consequently Erik missed some of his afternoon medications. The frenzied nurses spilled things and grew irritated with our request that they put blue food coloring into his feeding tube as had been the precautionary practice in the trauma unit. The colored liquid could be distinguished readily if the tube became dislodged and the liquid spilled out. The most alarming incident of the day occurred that evening, when Erik's feeding tube became dislodged and the Isotene, the liquid nutrition, started passing out of his nose. As Robert discovered this, one of the trauma unit nurses, who had fortunately stopped by as she was leaving the hospital from her shift, immediately began to suction the excess liquid from Erik's esophagus. There were no floor nurses around to observe this, for they were attending to patients in other rooms. Had we and the trauma unit nurse not been present, Erik could have drowned in his own liquid diet. This deeply unsettling event solidified our determination to stay with Erik and to hire private duty nurses as needed to assist with the medical aspects of his care.

Within one short but intense twelve-hour period our lives, which felt like Jeremian broken pots, were changing yet again. As we left the trauma unit as unceremoniously as we had come, trailing behind the pieces of equipment that held our son together, I realized that I had begun to feel protected by rising early, waiting sometimes patiently but more often anxiously in the foyer to the trauma unit, eating canned soup each night on the way "home" to our wounded community. Despite the struggle to secure information, to interpret medical discourse, to seek a human soul amidst the technological displays, we fought to hold our shattered son together. In the hallways, in the smoke-filled snack shop over our evening soup, in our Ronald McDonald House rollaway beds— along the margins of the world we glibly call normal—we turned the foreign into the familiar. In a world breaking apart literally and psychically, our young daughter's diary, our scribbled journals, and our memories screamed our longing for the return of a unified—though at present uncommunicative—brother and son. But beneath this hope, often hidden in the skirts of grief, lay hints of our separate, fragmented efforts simply to pay attention and to create some kind of connection with our "absent" son and brother that might sustain his life narrative.

Uncertain Deliveries

Where are you   going, my little one?
My little one,   where are you going today?
The short-handed   weekend staff
on seventh floor   did not resist
our presence   with Erik
nor the private duty   nurse watching
over him   the first two nights.

When the willful head nurse returned on Monday to find us with Erik as aides were performing bathing routines, she made her astonished displeasure amply clear. She huffed in and out of the room muttering against us disdainfully as we carefully cleared a path for her agitated movements. When Robert reported the feeding tube incident of Saturday evening she became immediately defensive, hearing in his words an attack on the competency of the medical staff. Witnessing a conflict that I knew could explode between the two of them within seconds, I tried to engage her calmly by reassuring her that the mishap had been inadvertent and a result of being short-staffed, not of incompetence. Though her tense facial muscles seemed to soften slightly as she turned and walked out of the room, I felt myself once again climbing onto the thread of fear and crawling away from pain and anger.

How like a battlefront the situation in which we found ourselves seemed as we adjusted to new surroundings, personnel, and routines. Although we were housed in the same hospital, we had changed arenas and faced new threats to our son. With fewer electronic monitoring devices attached to Erik to signal physical difficulties, without a nurse who was dedicated to observing him closely within a few yards, and with new regimens to learn, he was more exposed and vulnerable. As we remained, hour by hour and throughout shift changes, I felt bombarded by incongruities.

Chief among these was my realization that although this medical institution existed for the welfare of its patients, all of whom relied on it for their healing, they were often reduced to objects submissive to the will and convenience of the attending experts. Patients' voices and personal agency were disregarded as largely invisible decision makers manipulated their body parts and organs. The vocabulary and tone of voice with which many of the staff communicated to patients was frequently condescending or patronizing. When speaking together about particular patients, even in their presence, nurses and doctors relied on technical jargon that further objectified their patients. Even worse, they sometimes spoke pessimistically about patients' possibilities.

The treatment of Erik's roommate on the seventh floor became another example of troubling incongruities. Danny was a young man, older than Erik, who had sustained his severe brain injury in a motorcycle accident. When Erik moved into the room I noticed that Danny was alone in his half of the room. No one attended to or interacted with him regularly. Though the television was turned on, he registered no response to it nor could he call for any help. When the nurses periodically checked his IVs, urine bag, and feeding tube, they perfunctorily described what they were doing and occasionally plumped his pillows to adjust his drooping head. Danny's parents visited him only during regular evening visiting hours; sometimes on Sundays they brought the paper with them and sat reading in chairs against the wall at the foot of his bed. Discouraged from active participation in our children's care, I suspect that these parents also felt like interlopers in the medical world, just as we did.

In these circumstances I could not let go of a nagging question: who will represent those who cannot speak for themselves? Patients like Danny and Erik often receive the least attention because they cannot ring their call buttons. This common situation arises neither from medical maliciousness nor incompetence but from an interest in economics. Patient populations are too large to offer patients individualized care—the cost is deemed too high. Thoughts like this outraged me, for I was still trying to process the havoc wreaked, often on the innocent, by motor vehicular crashes. The compounded injustice of placing two comatose patients in the same room strengthened my determination to learn the languages that so thoroughly intimidate and separate patient from professional and deny the concerns of patients' families.

Having come of age during the Civil Rights movement and the nonviolent protests against the war in Vietnam, I gradually identified a vague similarity between the conviction that led people into the streets on behalf of justice and peace for people they did not know and our efforts to remain firmly but unobtrusively present with our injured son in a place where we were not welcome. From the Society of Friends and the Anabaptist religious tradition I had learned foremost to honor the principle of God moving my conscience and to question authorities demanding mindless obedience. Even though I regularly crawled away from conflict and fear or escaped into my head to avoid being overwhelmed by my feelings, I believed that if we could stay out of the professionals' way we could be of aid to our son, for whom any sense of future hung tenuously.

Despite the incongruities that swirled around us and the diminished patient-to-nurse ratio, we did gain a vastly extended amount of time to be with Erik. Even though we resented the higher priority given to economic profits than to patient needs, the deference paid to medical experts and the dismissive attitude toward parental concerns, and the adversarial tones that occasionally crept into conversations, we were determined to maintain a human link between our son and those on whom his survival still depended. Slowly we risked softening the adversarial atmosphere by trying to communicate with those whose territory we had entered. First we ventured simple smiles; then we expressed gratitude for ordinary things like changing IV bags or bed linens. Gradually we felt able to pose nonthreatening questions in order to learn better the language and assumptions of the seventh floor.

Through two trauma unit nurses who had given us their names and addresses in case we needed additional help, we quickly explored whether private duty nurses were permitted on the floor and whether the insurance company would pay for such services. During the first few days after Erik's transfer we hired highly recommended private duty nurses for the nighttime. As we became familiar with the floor routines and the personnel, my husband, my sister, and I rotated eight-hour shifts every twenty-four hours. All of us became adept at reading the remaining monitors and watching for peculiarities in the intravenous equipment; none of us had other patients, doctors, or reports to which to attend, so we read or talked to Erik, massaged and moved his limbs as we had watched the physical therapist do even before he left the trauma unit, and soothed him when he became restless.

The trauma unit physicians and the neurosurgeon continued to be Erik's doctors, though we still could not expect their appearance at any regular time or have much conversation with them. Since we were trying to piece together fragments of information about traumatic brain injury from nurses, from magazine articles on all kinds of subjects related to injuries and healing brought to us by friends, from respiratory and physical therapists who came daily to administer treatment to Erik and might drop a comment or two about changes in his lungs or his limbs, and from our own observations, I felt as people do when they are learning a foreign language and observing new cultural and social customs.

We always had many questions to ask the doctors, and we quickly found ourselves practicing the new terms or concepts we were picking up, hoping to enhance the medical professionals' willingness to communicate with us. My sister, husband, and I each assumed responsibility for posing the questions we had on our individual and common lists to any physician who might appear during our particular shift. We usually received indefinite answers. "No one can tell" was the standard, noncommittal response. Even though a few residents ventured a little more description of the range of outcomes we might expect—from a near vegetative state to a plateau of recovery that could occur at any point—we were left clutching our hope alone in a space filled with constant activity aimed theoretically at helping people heal.

Gradually, as I watched and talked with my unresponsive son hour by hour, I realized two things. First, had Erik received this injury just a few years earlier, he would not have survived. Though I did not fully appreciate on the day of Erik's injury the absolute necessity of speedy medical intervention when a traumatic brain injury occurs, I have since realized how crucial the first sixty minutes following the trauma are. Describing that "golden hour" and early, intensive interventions, William Winslade says that after the first hour "those systems left unaided tend to decline toward death or permanent damage to major organs."[1] Drawing on one study that "followed eighty-two brain-trauma patients with subdural hematomas—blood clots under the brain's tough outer layer," Winslade reports that "the mortality rate was 30 percent for those operated on within four hours of injury, 90 percent for those who waited longer."[2]

Damage and death occur not simply from mechanical damage to the brain but from delayed or secondary injuries that result from the brain's reaction to the injury. For example, if deprived of adequate oxygen, brain cells will begin to die within six minutes. Bleeding or blockage of air passages can cut off the oxygen supply. Also, when the bruised brain begins to swell and hits against the hard casing of the skull, pressure builds, further compromising the oxygen flow. In addition, the brain's chemical balance becomes chaotic after traumatic injury. "Because the brain regulates all physical functions essential to life, the victim may die or suffer permanent physical damage if the problem is not corrected quickly."[3] The kinds of intervention required for traumatic injuries—for example, airlifting victims to trauma center operating rooms, speedy surgeries to stop hemorrhaging or to repair damaged internal organs, adjusting chemical balances and monitoring pressure levels of the brain—were largely perfected during the Vietnam War. Ironically, medical techniques developed during a war we had protested were now prolonging our son's life.

The second thing I realized was that, despite the utility of these highly specialized treatments, even brain specialists could not predict how the brain would respond to radical interventions or how the entire organism would be affected by damage to the central control organ of the human body. Because the fear of litigation has been mounting for years in the medical profession, medical professionals walk a thin line between being circumspect and being routinely pessimistic. In those early weeks following Erik's injury I found myself emotionally incapable of absorbing the significance and potential implications of all the interventions that Erik experienced.

These dawning realities paradoxically increased my frustration and helplessness on the one hand, as on the other they pushed me toward some inner touchstone of resistance, even defiance, that turned my attention to watch for tiny changes rather than grand and global ones. On the first day of summer, an exquisitely clear June day, I began subliminally to recognize that we were on a journey that would not be finished at the end of summer. Fortunately for all of us, we could see only one day ahead as we kept track of our shifts and our questions and pursued our hearts' longing to forge some reconnective pathways to Erik.

With the start of summer vacation, Sonia spent two or three days each week with us at the hospital and the other days with Pat and Mike and other friends. She continued to record her observations in her diary, noting particularly hints of recovery and inexplicable signs that portended reversals.

Diary, I'm still down at the hospital and Erik is about the same. . . . To-
day we noticed that Erik opens his eyes like a blank stare and doesn't even
blink or anything. We have to touch him on the forehead to make him blink.
Dad's getting a little worried since Erik doesn't move his left leg. . . . We keep
talking to him and told him that it was the first day of summer!

During the fifth week Erik continued to open his eyes more frequently and spontaneously; sometimes we thought his eyes seemed even
to follow movements of our fingers or to be searching our faces. One day
when Sonia was present with us, she stood for a long time by Erik's bed
holding his hand. She spoke to him about all kinds of things, as she had
become fairly comfortable doing. On this particular day, however, she
was very eager to get him to respond to a direct request, something we
and other therapists had not been able to get him to do. Without explanation, Sonia focused her attention on his hand in making her request,
as if intuiting its significance to the brain's circuitry. Patiently she asked
Erik to move his little finger. Repeatedly she asked, rubbed the finger,
and then waited silently. Nothing. Then she spoke encouragingly a little more and asked again, sometimes almost taunting him to prove himself as siblings are accustomed to doing. Robert and I were both in the
room watching from the end of the bed. She asked another time, getting in front of Erik's face, and waited. Suddenly she exclaimed that
his finger had moved slightly. What to most observers would have been
imperceptible—and perhaps judged imagined—was for a little sister
and parents clinging to shreds of hope a giant step of reconnection within
Erik's body and between him and us.

The greater periods of wakefulness signaled a lightening of the coma
but certainly not the end of it. All my previous assumptions about coma
were challenged by our experience with Erik's traumatic brain injury.
Coma was not simply a clearly demarcated state of unconsciousness;
rather it was a changing, often fuzzy, state of unconsciousness. In many
patients coma does not end suddenly, as if turning on a light switch.
Though a coma usually means that the patient does not walk, talk, or
use his or her hands, sometimes even when unconscious a person may

move a limb or her head or make a noise. If a patient exhibits motor responses, eye opening, or vocal responses, one can assume that the coma is lifting. A rising score on the Glasgow Coma Scale indicates that the coma is lightening, although a patient may plateau for a period of time as he is emerging from a deep coma. In general, the shorter the duration of the coma, the better the long-term prognosis.

Almost simultaneously with longer periods of eye opening came undirected movement in other parts of Erik's body. He also exhibited periods of profound agitation when his face would contort, his eyes would fill with panic, and he would claw at the air or make weak attempts to roll back and forth in his bed. Because of his tracheostomy he could make no sounds, which must have compounded the sense of terror he was experiencing. During those times I crawled onto the bed with him and attempted to hold him calmly and to reassure him. Eventually the agitation would pass and he would fall exhausted into "sleep." Had we not been with him, physical restraints would have been placed on him for his own protection; we suspected that these would only have increased his agitation and impeded the speed, and possibly the extent, of his recovery.

As we witnessed these attacks of agitation we noticed that the right side of Erik's body was more active than the left; in fact, the left leg continued not to respond even to painful stimuli. One afternoon during my shift, while Erik was "napping," I sat beside his bed reading *The Healing Light,* a book given to me by a Quaker friend. As early as 1947 Agnes Sanford had described in this little book an innate potential for healing that resides in the human being and becomes available as one learns to respect and practice the spiritual laws that govern this aspect of the divine-human relationship. Because I was learning to communicate through the body with my son, I was very interested in Sanford's descriptions of the potential for healing through God's laws of faith and love. As I read on, I gently and rather mindlessly placed my hand on Erik's left leg, at first simply continuing to read. And then I stopped reading and turned my attention to the physical sensation of his leg under my hand. I found myself visualizing or meditating on the intricate network of muscles, veins, nerves, and ligaments running throughout his entire body. Then I considered my own willingness to be a kind of conduit through which any healing energy I might have could pass through to him. Gradually I became aware of a great warmth on my hand, and I very lightly moved my hand over the length of his leg. I experienced peace and gratitude for this quiet time, this nonverbal communication with Erik.

As had become our usual pattern now, Sharon took the shift from 11:00 P.M. until 7:00 A.M. Throughout the night when Erik seemed "awake" Sharon played music on a small tape recorder, talked with him, and read novels. At this particular time she had been reading C. S. Lewis's *Prince Caspian* to him. When I'd been home for Sonia's birthday party I had taken it from his bookshelf for this purpose. Since he had read it a few years earlier, I thought hearing it in the recesses of unconsciousness might arouse memory in him. Each night Sharon's animated reading invited Erik, from a lost "realm" we could not enter, to travel into the enchanted stories of Dr. Cornelius, tutor of Prince Caspian. The following morning I came in to relieve Sharon from her night-shift journey to Narnia. Her big news was that Erik had moved his left leg a little during the night; she urged me to watch for that during the day to see if it continued. Until then I had not told anyone about my previous day's experience while reading *The Healing Light,* but then I did. We began to watch the slow return of movement to a leg that had been virtually paralyzed.

We were now in the third week on the seventh floor—the sixth week since the accident. Each day's routines were interrupted and enriched by visitors or gifts of flowers, cards, books, or posters made by classmates to hang on the wall. Erik's adviser from school came regularly and brought with her other favorite teachers. Members from the Friends Meeting offered to sit with Erik for an hour or two in the afternoons so that we could leave the hospital for a little while. The Friend who had delivered that startling, brief message in worship at about the time Erik was being injured—"No one knows how long he will live"—brought him a tape recording of Tibetan monks chanting. Many voices united in one resonant sound reverberated across centuries and bathed Erik's room and grounded his body in primal sound. With that small gift our Friend brought the tonal basis of the universe, expressed through an ancient tradition from a distant culture, into Erik's presence. To Erik's friends who sent inquiries and cards via the teachers, and who were going their separate ways for the summer, we returned this basic message: "Love each other, care for each other, appreciate what you have when you have it, and join us in holding hope for Erik's healing."

One of the visits we had arranged at the recommendation of our Princeton pediatrician, and anticipated with hope and anxiety, occurred about three weeks after Erik had moved to the seventh floor. Dr. Derek Bruce, a pediatric neurosurgeon from the University of Pennsylvania, had agreed to come to Cooper Hospital in Camden, look over the CT scans and medical records, and observe Erik. We did not want the Cooper physicians to feel that we were ungrateful for their work, but we wanted to ascertain whether everything was being done that possibly could be to encourage the best outcome for Erik. From the outset we had to weigh trade-offs in Erik's treatment. For example, although a small town or suburban hospital like Princeton's might have been more friendly and comfortable for us, it would not have had the experience in treating traumatic brain injuries that Camden did. Now we compared the treatment record of Camden with the value of research into brain function and capacities that is routinely part of a university hospital.

Because he was not personally invested in this case, or perhaps simply by nature of his personality, Dr. Bruce was warmly humane toward us and Erik. He exuded professional competence and confidence as he examined Erik, performed tests on him that had become familiar, and asked us questions about what we had been doing and witnessing. Although he emphasized the severity of Erik's injury, acknowledged the then current assumption that injured brain cells do not rejuvenate, and stressed the unpredictability of how the brain might establish new connections where old pathways had been damaged, he also indicated that Erik's age, excellent physical condition, and high I.Q. worked to his advantage in this crisis. Asserting that the more one takes into brain trauma the more one is likely to have after the trauma, he reminded us of what we had recently read in some brain injury literature—that we couldn't safely predict an outcome until at least six months to a year had passed. Since 1985 those time frames have been significantly revised, so that now we recognize that people with severe brain injuries may continue to change one, two, or more years following the injury.

Dr. Bruce's visit lifted our spirits enormously, not because he made any promises but because he discussed Erik's injuries in the context of Erik's personal biography. Both a neurosurgeon and a pediatrician, he perceptively combined discrete details from Erik's medical history with an understanding of Erik as a child trapped inside chaos and struggle. His manner was nonthreatening to the Camden trauma doctors, one of whom participated in Dr. Bruce's examination of Erik. Indeed, Dr. Bruce's knowledge of a child's developing brain, its cognitive malleability, and the greater relative resiliency of youth for healing seemed to encourage the Camden medical staff as well. Though nothing had changed in Erik during Dr. Bruce's consultation, the opportunity simply to have a neurosurgeon speak with us about a whole person—our son—offered us the first real, external hope we had had since May 26.

Shortly following Dr. Bruce's visit Erik's physicians and a hospital social worker advised us to begin looking for a rehabilitation institution to which we could send Erik. Just as the seventh floor personnel and regimens became familiar, we were forced to contemplate another frontier. Our lives were so tightly tied to the daily routines of the seventh floor that I had not considered what would happen next. I guess I assumed we would stay there until Erik "got well" and we could go home. Even with the enduring severity of our child's injury facing us every day, and buoyed by Dr. Bruce's visit, I lived still trying to reach behind the injury to our son—that presence of a whole being who was alive in my memory and imagination—and sometimes I was nearly oblivious to the meaning and long-term consequences of his condition. As professionals explained that he would need much more intensive therapy—physically, cognitively, socially—than any acute care hospital could provide, I found myself again defiantly crawling away from my feelings.

Almost simultaneous with the dropped hint that Erik would need prolonged, additional treatment beyond the acute care hospital, Erik's physical therapist recommended trying to transport him from his room to the therapy room in another part of the hospital, where he could put Erik on the tilting table to see how his heart rate and blood pressure would respond to being upright after lying in a prone position for six weeks. The transport alone was a challenge, for Erik became easily agitated at any movement. He had to be tied into the wheelchair to keep from falling out, and he needed the reassurance of physical touch and virtually constant, quiet speaking close to his head, as we proceeded through the hallways and into elevators.

While monitoring Erik's blood pressure and pulse closely, the therapist slowly raised the table to 45 degrees, left it there for several minutes, and then brought the table back to a flat position. Then he raised it again a few degrees higher. On this first occasion Erik tolerated the changes in elevation satisfactorily. After the session, however, he seemed exceedingly worn out, and he fell into a deeper sleep or level of coma for the next day. During this period, the neurosurgeon ordered another routine CT scan and reported that the subdural hygroma was a tiny bit larger on this new scan than on the scan taken nine days earlier. A subdural hygroma is a cystic swelling, or sac of fluid, that occurs in the thin membrane of the brain between the tough, fibrous membrane that encloses the brain and spinal cord and the more delicate, vasculated membrane that adheres to the brain and carries blood to and from the cerebral cortex. The neurosurgeon suggested that Erik's increased sleepiness could be a result of pressure from further accumulating cerebral fluid, and therefore he might need to drain the area again. He advised a wait-and-see attitude, but if draining were necessary again—suggesting that this condition might continue to recur—he might recommend inserting a shunt that would allow the excess fluid to drain from the cerebral cavity.

As we assumed a watchful stance toward this potentially threatening development we experienced a profound pull in sometimes contradictory directions: remaining close to our son, and visiting rehabilitation centers. Increased activity around Erik held us like magnets to his side. Therapeutic interventions became more frequent and intense as Erik's body responded to stimuli. Bedside physical therapy was replaced by demanding and exhausting trips to the physical therapy section of the hospital. For six weeks Erik's only nutrition had come through a feeding tube. Now instructions came to let Erik have chips of ice occasionally so the speech therapist could observe the condition of his tongue activity and swallowing reflexes. Would he be able to move small ice chips with his tongue and to swallow? The respiration therapist appeared more frequently, and the neurosurgeons talked of doing an EEG to examine brain activity and patterns. The flurry of activity made us want to be engaged as much as possible as participant-witnesses of these interventions.

Indeed, because Erik could tolerate a 70-degree angle of elevation on the tilting table and because his movements in bed were increasing, the physical therapist suggested that we and the nurses move him to a chair beside the bed for a few minutes each day. At first transferring him from the bed to the chair was like moving a puppet whose limbs are held together by strings. Erik had no control over any part of his body; we had to move every piece of him. When he was in the chair he could not hold himself erect but needed to be leaned against the back of the chair and supported on either side to prevent him from flopping over sideways or sliding frontward out of the chair. During this initial change of position, which lasted only a few minutes, Erik became very agitated. But each subsequent day his agitation lessened, and his ability to hold his upper body upright strengthened. One day he launched into a kind of forward and backward rocking motion. As I squatted on the floor by his chair to be at eye level with him, he fell forward with his arms outstretched. Robert grabbed him and held him for a moment and then helped him move backward in the chair. There were tears in his and our eyes as we told him how much we loved him. In the midst of this movement, one of the trauma unit physicians dropped by and exclaimed, "My God, he's trying to hug you." That was the first time one of our Camden medical professionals had overtly acknowledged Erik as a person or attributed intention to this being they had been probing and photographing and treating for over a month. Had no one been present, these motions most likely would have been missed; if observed only by detached medical personnel, they might have been regarded as random and purposeless.

This lurching forward and reaching out became a pattern, repeated again and again, with Erik laying his head on our shoulders for a few seconds, especially as he was moved from his bed to a chair. Robert, who was close to Erik and strong enough not to be overpowered by his unpredictable physical movements, assisted all such transfers. Robert could be gentle in preventing Erik from getting hurt while allowing him to move, thereby gaining physical strength and perhaps making new motor connections in the brain.

In the midst of these daily events the hospital staff advised us to go out and investigate another unfamiliar world, the world of rehabilitation centers. The hospital social worker frequently brought recommendations about rehabilitation facilities that we should consider, and she offered to make appointments for us. For a few days we put her off, saying that there were too many things happening with Erik at that point; we couldn't take off to make yet another accommodation to the world of traumatic brain injury. She persisted, against our resistance, to push us beyond the second-stage "security" of the acute care hospital. We deeply longed to be free of hospitals and considered in private the possibility of just taking Erik home, away from all medical directives, and trying to establish our own care program, so great was our yearning to return life to some semblance of familiarity, even as our recognition that nothing would ever be the same again continued to deepen.

We finally relented to the pressure of the social worker after surveying the opinions of the doctors and therapists involved in Erik's care. Our condition for arranging appointments with various rehabilitation institutions was that we would hire a private duty nurse during our hours away and insofar as possible not schedule appointments on days that Erik was scheduled for major tests or trips to the physical therapy department.

Over the next two or three weeks the tension between staying close to Erik and traveling to Pennsylvania, Delaware, and various points in New Jersey—not to mention hours spent in telephone conversations with other rehabilitation facilities and the fledgling National Head Injury Foundation—led to an enlarged conversation. Whereas in the trauma unit and during the first two weeks on the seventh floor we tried to stay in close communication with Erik's body and soul, we were now forced to master new information to function as liaisons between his injured state of being and the world of rehabilitation on which he and we would need to depend. Spiderlike, I attentively wove my web between what was going on with Erik at the hospital and what Robert and I were discovering as we visited rehabilitation facilities.

Despite the insistence with which the social worker had advised and arranged for appointments at two highly recommended rehabilitation centers, no one had prepared us for what we would find in the larger world of rehabilitation. In both centers we were greeted politely but perfunctorily. We sat in small social worker offices, listening to the services their respective institutions could provide. In neither case did the social worker refer to our son by name, even when asking questions about his current condition. No one inquired about who he had been at the time of his injury or anything about the circumstances of the accident. We offered that information, but it was not sought. When we were taken on a tour of the facilities I was outraged to find a dormlike room with several beds holding human bodies in various stages of alertness. Erik would take one of these beds if he were to come here. There was one nurse, working on the edge of the room with charts and medicines, who was responsible for these eight beds of patients. In the background a television droned and flashed blotches of animated color onto the walls and fixed eyes of these children and young people. The unattractive, uncongenial therapy rooms were also depressing. I was simply unprepared to enter a world in which the maimed, gathered together, were totally dependent on the good faith and will of those who had trained to help them restore their lives. In my own state of vulnerability I was shocked by how mechanical all the interactions seemed. Weights, bicycles, steps, and parallel bars filled the therapy room. Some kind of rock music filled the air to stimulate or distract or confuse. What, I wondered to myself, if someone here has different musical preferences?

As we left the first site Robert and I tried to encourage each other despite the alarm that was resounding in us. This center was undergoing some renovations, which may have made optimal conditions and patient service difficult. The next place, we hoped, would be better. To be sure, the next center was not being remodeled, but our reception was similar to that in the first. The public relations skills of the second facility's social worker fortunately surpassed the first's, for she clearly and quickly communicated the relevant features of their program. But she also was not interested in knowing our son personally, leading me to leap to the conclusion that impersonality would be a characteristic of the rehabilitation world. I assumed that people would be known by their disability and functional improvements, not by some psychological-spiritual capacity for meaning-making. At neither of these two rehabilitation centers were family members urged to participate in therapies; they were simply to be available to take patients for home visits when appropriate. Sonia accompanied us on these two visits and later recorded her own astute observations.

Diary, . . . Mom, Dad, and I went to visit some rehab. places today. The looks weren't very appealing except for the ocean and boardwalk bit. We met the social worker and the occupational therapist. They had some nice stuff but it was just depressing and gloomy. I couldn't imagine Erik going there. Mom came home and got sick. She said it was hard.

When we returned to the parking garage of Cooper Hospital at the end of the day I had a severe headache accompanied by nausea. I had been rendered virtually speechless from what I had witnessed.

Over subsequent days we made additional phone calls to collect more information, and Robert visited other facilities by himself as I remained at the hospital. Between visits to rehabilitation centers, we accompanied Erik to his physical therapy sessions and continued our bedside activities with an occupational therapist, who came more regularly to try to elicit purposeful responses from him.

As moving Erik between the bed and the chair and the bed and the wheelchair to transport him to the therapy room for the tilting table exercises became part of our daily routine, we observed two changes. First, he began almost frantically to resist going into the wheelchair. Second, he started putting weight on his legs as if to help himself to move even though his total lack of coordination prevented this. On July 1 the physical therapist elevated the tilting table to 80 degrees. Erik became extremely agitated at that elevation, but his blood pressure remained stable. When the therapist lowered the table, he placed Erik's feet on the floor and waited to see what Erik might do. With Robert on one side and the therapist supporting on the other, Erik began to take wobbling steps. He took not one or two steps, as the therapist had anticipated, but began to stagger across the therapy room, his limbs gangling like a scarecrow's, his head stuffed with tangled neural nets. All activity in the therapy room stopped as therapists and clients watched amazed. When he had gone halfway across the room, spontaneous applause broke out as Robert and I embraced our severely altered son with tears of incredible joy. Though Erik's score on the Glasgow Coma Scale had risen from the low of 3 to perhaps 6 on some days, Erik was still considered to be in a coma, for he had no vocal response and could not respond to commands.

Daily over the next two weeks new staff came to work with Erik or new equipment appeared. Observing Erik's interest in pulling himself up in bed by using one of our arms for stable support, we inquired about attaching a trapeze bar overhead that he might use at his initiative. Within a day or two one was installed, and we began the tedious task of constructing a path of repetition-communication between his body, his brain, and the bar. Though there may have been no causal connection, only a coincidental one, Dr. Bruce's visit two weeks previous had not only offered us strands of hope but also apparently activated the medical staff and rehabilitation personnel in the hospital to treat Erik more aggressively.

The significance of this second-opinion consultation combined with our determination to stay engaged in our son's care forced me eventually to acknowledge the privilege our employers afforded us. I say eventually because much of the time in the first six weeks I paid little attention to what other patients and their families were doing. Because I worked on an academic schedule and did not teach summer school, I could easily lay aside my own research project to remain at the hospital. Robert's employer generously urged him to stay with Erik week after week. As our vigil stretched toward July and as we met other family members coming for brief visiting periods, I also recognized the consequences of social and economic inequities for the severely injured.

The injustice of such inequities was confirmed poignantly for us one day as we carried out our usual activities and storytelling around Erik's bed. His comatose roommate, whose human contact was limited to evening visits from his parents and the minimal care of nurses, treatment by the respiration therapist to prevent pneumonia, and once-daily manipulation of his limbs by a physical therapist, had shown no signs of responsiveness for weeks prior to Erik's arrival in the room. One morning as an aide came to prepare Danny for his bath she exclaimed, "My God, look, Danny's head has moved." It had turned to face toward the human interaction occurring on Erik's side of the room. Though this was observed by two or three nurses, I witnessed no increased effort to build on this small indication of response. What was written in Danny's case notes that day? Did anyone inform his parents? In another room a few doors away the young girl who had been thrown from a horse and had arrived in the trauma unit just a few days after Erik was also struggling without much familial support. Though the families of Danny and the young girl were conforming to hospital expectations, no doubt out of necessity, not preference, I was outraged about the human costs born from such inequities and from the deference paid to medical authority. Were there not people who could companion these young lives on their confusing journeys, I wondered repeatedly. What were the stories Danny might benefit from hearing? What were his fears? His loves? Who could give them voice to and for him?

Growing increasingly uncertain after many phone calls and visits about whether we would find a rehabilitation facility adequate to meet Erik's needs, Robert and Sonia and I drove to Wilmington, Delaware, to visit the Alfred I. Dupont Children's Hospital. We had learned about this institution from some friends whose daughter, born with spina bifida many years earlier, had been treated there over the years by an outstanding pediatrician. Preliminary inquiries revealed that though the hospital had a traumatic brain injury unit it was young and small. We acknowledged that this lack of experience could be a disadvantage. The medical rehabilitation facility itself was new and inviting. After announcing ourselves, we waited in an airy, spacious, colorful lobby for the director of the traumatic brain injury unit. Barbara McHugh arrived quickly and, sitting down with us, greeted us warmly. Immediately she acknowledged how difficult we must be finding this process and then turned to our thirteen-year-old daughter. "Tell me," she said, "about your brother." This was only the second time in six weeks that Erik's personhood had been initially acknowledged by a medical professional, despite his tenuous balance between life and death. McHugh asked us questions about his interests, his special abilities, his school and friends, our feelings, his current condition. In this brief conversation our own humanity and feelings were respected. Following these preliminaries we toured the brain injury unit, meeting nurses and therapists, observing therapies in session, and learning about the unit's philosophy of rehabilitation. There were no dorm-style rooms, but a combination of private and semiprivate rooms; each patient received a primary care nurse who followed the patient's care throughout the duration of the patient's stay. Though the director assured us that they could and would give Erik the highest-quality care without our vigilance, she did not discourage our interest in participating regularly in his therapies. By the time we returned to Camden and Cooper Hospital that evening all three of us had reached an inward decision about where to continue treatment when the time came. The final stage of our decision to go to the Dupont Hospital occurred when Barbara McHugh came to Camden to assess Erik's needs in relation to Dupont's facilities.

Erik's release from Cooper Hospital depended on the completion of an EEG and the condition of the subdural hygroma. A delicate task under the best of conditions, performing the EEG on a restless, still comatose brain-injured teenager who could not understand what had happened to him was a major challenge. As we did for every test, scan, or surgery, we patiently narrated what would happen or was happening to Erik. Trying to keep him calm, we explained that all the wires attached to his head would help the doctors check for seizure activity and monitor the progression to more normal brain waves. We hoped that the recent aggressive therapies and Erik's increased responsiveness to stimuli indicated a lessening of the intracranial pressure. On the day before our scheduled departure from Cooper Hospital the CT scan revealed that although the brain ventricles were still enlarged, they were in a nearly normal position, suggesting, the neurosurgeon reported, a reabsorption of cerebral fluid. The way forward to yet another world opened before us.

On the morning of the high summer day that Erik would be taken by ambulance to Dupont, I arrived at 7:30 A.M. to find Erik dressed in clean pajamas for his trip. Sharon and Carol, his private duty nurse, had narrated the day's approaching events as they quietly bathed and dressed him. Though still alternating between periods of agitation and calm, Erik was resting peacefully when I entered his room. The occupational therapist came in once more to check Erik's responsiveness. She rang small bells that she wanted Erik to stop, and then bounced a tennis ball for which she hoped he might reach. To our delight, he responded to both these exercises for the first time. In my journal of that last morning I recorded the following:

At 9:30 Robert and Erik took off for Wilmington in the ambulance. Sonia, Sharon, and I ate breakfast in the midst of tears and laughter, then went back to the Ronald McDonald House to pack and load the car and clean the room. . . .

It is difficult to say farewell to people who have helped Erik a great deal during his time at Cooper. Although I am glad to leave Camden and Cooper, I leave behind a large part of my thankful heart, broken for my son and for others like Danny who remain struggling. . . .

These words, as I record them now, evoke feelings in my body cells as if I'd made this momentous move just last week. What is this remarkable capacity called memory that inhabits our entire bodies?

What I longed for at the time of this transition was some kind of marking to place on our path or some ritual that would help us convey the significance of all that had transpired in our lives in this decaying American city. I left some notes and said farewells, but in the end we appeared to walk out of the medical narrative as impersonally as we had come into it. It would continue to be enacted by new characters whose conditions would be described in case notes by doctors.

When we left the medical world for the rehabilitation world I was immersed simply in living the day-to-day experiences and in trying to assimilate in my own brain all that was occurring. I did not reflect systematically on what the medical narrative had taught us. Only retrospectively have I realized the extent to which I was conceiving Erik's journey through brain injury as a narrative. As I reached into the profound silence of coma with words and images, I was attempting to weave a story from chaos that might help Erik and us eventually hobble toward meaning.

I recognized from the outset of this dreadful journey that our experience of reality and the ways our lives seemed to cohere had been violently assaulted by the accident. Gradually I discovered how sharply our lived personal stories—which were sustained by multiple subplots, extended across generations, laced with symbols, and filtered through our values—were shattered and ignored by the medical world. Despite their vocation as healers, the medical personnel held a far narrower and more mechanistic view of reality than ours. Faced with this alarming realization, I learned quickly that for Erik's survival we would find a way to bridge the gaps in language between our personal stories and the medical ones and to mitigate the adversarial tension between the two styles of discourse and their purposes. As I reflect over the intervening years since our departure from the acute care hospital, I perceive with greater clarity what we learned from medical discourse.

Through anguish and blundering, we discovered in rudimentary form the ways the human brain afflicted by injury reacts. This invisible organ, which I had taken for granted to direct my movement and basic survival as well as my highly abstract cogitation, I now investigated with simultaneous curiosity, anxiety, and gratitude. Without any experience in neuroscience, we learned that an individual may have a head injury without having a brain injury, and we learned the difference between a closed head injury (when there is no break in the skull) and an open head injury. On the first day the trauma doctors had explained the difference between a focal brain injury—an injury isolated to a specific spot or section of the brain—and a diffuse injury that affects multiple parts of the brain. Erik's diffuse injury was caused by the assault of the crash, which forced the brain to bump around inside the skull.

From the moment the bolt was inserted in Erik's skull we began to learn about the role of cerebrospinal fluid, which maintains a positive pressure called intracranial pressure (I.C.P.). A rise in the I.C.P. above 18 to 20 cms in a brain-injured patient usually signals either cerebral edema (swelling of the brain) or intracranial hemorrhage (bleeding inside the skull), which is considered a delayed or secondary hemorrhage.

When the neurosurgeon recommended surgery to relieve what he suspected was a collection of spinal fluid inside the skull putting pressure on the ventricles, we simply accepted his advice. Later I grasped how the coverings of the brain—technically called the meninges, made up of the dura mater, the pia mater, and the arachnoid mater—hold the brain hammock-like inside the skull and keep it from swinging too much from one side to the other. Between each of these linings there is a layer of fluid that assists in maintaining the balance of the brain inside the skull. After injuries like Erik's, cystlike sacs of serous fluid, called hygromas or hematomas, can form between these layers and prolong coma and further threaten the brain.

By looking at CT scans and crude sketches of the brain in photocopied articles passed to us by caring friends, I constructed a picture of the brain in my imagination so that I could conceptualize its organization. By witnessing over six weeks the very gradual "arising" of responsiveness in Erik's organism, I intuited the evolutionary and hierarchical character of the brain from the fish brain to the reptilian brain to the mammalian brain to the human cortex, I also understood from our close attention to and interactions with Erik that each of these "layers" of the brain has sensory input and motor output functions that are peculiar to it but dependent upon the functioning of the lower levels. Indeed, consciousness had to return in a conelike channel, through each layer of the brain, beginning at the smallest point with such primal mechanisms as respiration and blood pressure and moving onward to the control of movement in the limbs and torso and eventually to the highly discriminatory functions carried on by the human cortex. By the time we left Cooper Hospital, Erik's fish and reptilian brains were responding in ways that gave us encouragement.

In mid-July 1985, when we left Cooper Hospital, the prevailing view of traumatic brain injury in the medical narrative was that there was little one could do to affect the outcome, which was generally presented as pessimistic. We defied the repeated invitations to leave his bedside and to get on with our own lives and the accusations of medical professionals and social workers alike that we were unable to come to terms with the reality and consequences of the automobile crash. Instead, the more closely we watched and related to Erik, even without his apparent responsiveness, the more we became convinced that one does not become a self the first time—or a second time—alone. Looking back to July 1985, two months after the accident, I realize that as we left Cooper Hospital in Camden we were struggling with conflicting views of reality. Although we had read about Prince Caspian, his betraying uncle King Miraz, Dr. Cornelius, and the magical kingdom governed by Aslan, the noble lion, simply to surround Erik with language sounds and narrative structures, I was struck subsequently by the provocative analogies between Narnia and the mysterious, enigmatic world of coma. Indeed, the stories of Narnia opened me to the magical qualities of our relationship with our injured child and of all living organisms.

In Lewis's Narnia series, four highly imaginative English children move between the visible world of English society and boarding school and an invisible, magical kingdom governed by a noble lion and filled with walking trees, talking beasts, and dwarves. Each of the books in the Narnia series chronicles threats from would-be usurpers or those fearful of enchantment and describes arduous obstacles like malevolent witches, lost trails, dense woods, and deep waters that must be confronted before the protagonists can return to Narnia.

The narrative in *Prince Caspian* moves in two directions simultaneously: in one Caspian faces repeated obstructions and bodily challenges as he flees the pursuing troops of his uncle, who threatens to wipe out memory; in the second, the royal children, who are inwardly compelled to reach Caspian and offer him their assistance, try to follow the circuitous and torturous path leading toward him, and they too encounter momentous obstacles. Resolution occurs only as the stories these two groups remember and retell converge, and memory partakes of reality. The flight, confusion, wooded dead-ends, paths that circle back on themselves, and undecipherable voices coming from unseen hills all metaphorically suggest the arduous path of trying to re-story one's life after brain injury.

Unarticulated questions lurked beneath the surface of our nighttime reading. Could we help to reawaken or to reforge memory lines in body cells and in neural paths? Would Erik gradually be able to produce non-verbal images of the sensory and motor systems in "conversation" with an interactive—even enchanted, if you will—world of time and space?

Could such activities eventually be clothed in language that would enable Erik to have a restored sense of his own subjectivity and permit him
to take up his own narrative?

In the daylight Robert and I constantly asked other, more rudimentary, questions. Robert's were graphic and anguished. Will he ever get
out of bed and into a wheelchair and walk alone? Will he ever know
who he is? Will he ever know I am his father? Will he ever again have
a girlfriend? be able to marry? be able to have children? be able to earn
a living? Though I also harbored Robert's questions, I was, perhaps because of my personality or my fear of the answers, inclined to stay close
to the present and to attend directly to Erik's struggling being. In the
midst of sometimes radically different views of reality, I wondered
whether there was anything commensurate between the assumptions
made by medical professionals about reality for the brain injured and
the reality embodied in Erik's biographical-familial story. I carried that
question inside me as I followed the ambulance south on I-95 to the rehabilitation world. Understanding after seven weeks that our son would
not in an instant be well or return to "normal," I now wondered what
the next course on this journey would show us.

THRESHOLD FOUR

Becoming Again

The day	that Erik wobbled
halfway	across the therapy room
held up on either side	by father and a therapist,
something in me	quickened as if
new life	had stirred.

Erik left Cooper Hospital, accompanied by his father, in an ambulance headed south toward Wilmington, Delaware, on a morning in mid-July. Their trip to the Dupont Children's Hospital recalled the yet-unborn child's journey through the birth canal. Robert had indirectly participated in Erik's first birth by lovingly coaching me during a long labor; in this second "birth," he directly supported and conveyed our son toward fuller consciousness.

Because Erik inclined easily to agitation at this stage, medical personnel and the ambulance company permitted Robert to ride beside Erik. We believed Robert's presence would be comforting to Erik and would eliminate the need for restraints, which we thought would only heighten his agitation, and spare him from possible sedation. All of us had prepared ourselves and Erik for his departure. Over the preceding two or three days we had expressed our gratitude in Erik's presence to therapists, nurses, and doctors as part of saying farewell and as preparation for the next phase of the story.

Every mile of the way Robert explained to Erik what was happening. "Now we're going to get on the elevator and go downstairs, where the ambulance is waiting." When they emerged into the July air Robert asked, "Do you feel how warm it is this morning? Can you feel the breeze on your face? It's been a long time since you've been outside. It must feel pleasant." As attendants settled Erik in the cavern of the ambulance, father moved close to son, speaking soothingly, "Soon we'll be on the way."

In the ambulance Robert sat close to Erik, who reclined throughout the trip. The even, reassuring tones of Robert's voice accompanied the sound of the ambulance motor, carrying them together backward and forward in the present. The trip was long. To fill the time Robert began again to tell Erik about our relatives and friends and about their love for him. He affirmed Erik's many fine qualities, creating with them a litany: determination, honesty, patience, kindness, intelligence, compassion, tolerance, integrity. Robert also charted their progress on the road and linked present conditions to memories. "The sky is really clear blue today. It would be a good day for baseball. Remember when we went to the Mets game? You have been one of their most loyal fans, even though they haven't been doing so well this season. Do you remember your Little League days? I always enjoyed getting to your games. You were quite a good second baseman. Do you remember the summer you and Steve and Dave built the tree house? How hard you all worked! There sure is a lot of construction on this road, but it looks like traffic is moving along. . . . If you want to sleep just close your eyes. I'll stay right here beside you. You have been through so much and have come a long way these past seven weeks. Just rest now." Throughout the journey such expression of love supported Erik's slow, still uncertain, passage from the womb of coma to independent life.

When Sonia, Sharon, and I arrived at Dupont Children's Hospital about an hour and a half behind the ambulance, we found Erik resting peacefully in a pleasant private room with a large window that let in natural light and overlooked the outside grounds. The young woman who would be his primary nurse was attentively gathering additional information from Robert about Erik and his history. All the rooms on the traumatic brain injury unit opened onto a wide "nerve" center, where therapists and medical staff communicated and recorded their case notes. Around this open circle were several alcoves for visiting in groups or for watching television. My first impression was that we had entered a well-attended, mindful, unhurried environment. And despite all the new people and routines that awaited us, I relaxed momentarily.

As we were preparing for the transition to Dupont, a move that took us another 60 miles farther away from our home, we had inquired about other Ronald McDonald facilities and wondered how we would be able to maintain our own lives and our connection to Erik's care without such a place. Through the thoughtfulness of friends we became the houseguests of Fred and Winnie Hoover, our friends' aunt and uncle. At the outset neither they nor we considered that we would remain more than a few nights, until we found our way in this new place. But their mercy and concern welcomed us to stay longer each time we suggested moving elsewhere.

The transition to the rehabilitation facility brought my sister's departure. She had been with us for five weeks, so saying farewell to her just two days after we arrived at Dupont not only was extremely difficult but also represented palpably the enduring nature of the changes that had befallen us. We would need to continue our lives, with the uncertainties and impairments that were becoming real to us, as a family of four.

During the first two days at Dupont we were assimilated slowly into the routines of the traumatic brain injury rehabilitation unit. One by one the medical director, an intern or two, the speech, physical, and occupational therapists, the neurologist, and, several days later, the psychologist came by Erik's room to introduce themselves and to discuss their roles in Erik's rehabilitation plan. Each therapist made the initial assessments of Erik's condition necessary to chart a treatment plan. As early as the first day of Erik's arrival, the head of the speech therapy department came to observe Erik's tongue and chewing actions and swallowing reflexes as she fed him his soft diet. The following day the physical therapist came for him and wheeled him to an airy, colorful therapy room that opened through glass doors onto an outer courtyard, where some therapies could also be conducted. Staff members were careful to introduce Erik and us to other patients, despite Erik's inability to acknowledge anyone else.

One of the first differences we experienced between the medical and rehabilitation worlds was that all patients were dressed in their own street clothes at the rehabilitation center. Even though some young people spent a significant amount of time resting in their beds, they were not permitted to remain in pajamas or hospital gowns. Though Erik was still in a light coma and therefore may not have recognized the difference between a hospital gown and Ocean Pacific shorts and a polo shirt, I was shocked to see a shell of our former son in familiar clothes that used to fit him well and now dangled from his body.

Just as a newborn infant comes into the world naked and alone, needing to be outfitted with clothes that enable him or her to live in the new environment, so Erik arrived at Dupont, needing to be habilitated both to the regimen of rehabilitation and, eventually, for society. To rehabilitate him meant to clothe him again with movement—crawling, walking, balancing, running; to clothe him with habits of self-care like eating and eliminating in socially appropriate ways; to clothe him with language and cognition and social skills. While parents of newborns await these developments with confidence, we wondered if they would all be possible now a second time. In short, the rehabilitation world would describe Erik's condition, including his needs, abilities, and deficits, in ways that would create a dwelling in which he might live and relate to the outside world.

The careful deliberateness with which the staff welcomed Erik into the routines of Dupont led in a few days to a comforting regular, though dynamic, rhythm. The combination of private and semiprivate rooms gave us the privilege of staying overnight with him and made visitation comfortable and relatively unintrusive on others' needs or desires for quiet. The wide hallways offered ample space for the movement of wheelchairs and beds. An array of courtyards, several with lovely fountains, gave patients the stimulation of the out-of-doors in protected areas. The gardenlike grounds around the hospital offered patients and their families places to walk or sit in warm summer and fall weather. Each patient's primary nurse coordinated his or her treatment plan and therapy schedule. Erik received two sessions daily of speech, physical, and occupational therapies. During the first days some of these therapies were conducted in his room.

The sense of balance or harmony—what I refer to as rhythm— reflected significant differences between the medical world we had just left and the rehabilitation world we had entered. Almost from the beginning of our association with the Dupont Children's Hospital we recognized that, in the discourse of rehabilitation, multiple narrators would plot and interpret Erik's treatment story. What we would discover over the three months we spent at Dupont were the assumptions and underlying philosophies about injury, disability, and rehabilitation that governed the overarching narrative.

In the rehabilitation setting, injury, which had consumed us for seven weeks, receded to history. This became clear to us when the medical director and pediatrician did not appear immediately upon Erik's arrival. Within the short space of half a day we had left a medical environment focused on crisis intervention and entered the realm of disability. Now nurses made preliminary assessments and presumably wrote those in case notes that the various medical specialists then read. Throughout Erik's residency at Dupont the medical staff remained more on the periphery, addressing residual or secondary problems like removing trachea tubes or gastrointestinal feeding lines and monitoring neurological changes that might signal a delayed reaction in the brain to the original traumatic event.

Therapists, social workers, and psychologists became the main actors to usher Erik into the language and experience of disability. Though each therapist's personality, life stage, and experience influenced the character of his or her interactions with Erik, all regarded disabilities in general as conditions to be assimilated into one's life or to which one must adapt with compensatory strategies. Despite their generally optimistic outlooks, their enthusiasm to assist patients regain lost capacities, and their professionalism in developing alternative physical or cognitive approaches, no one guided Erik, or us as his parents, through the gap between the realm of his earlier vibrant capability and the kingdom of his present disability. No one could hear the thoughts riveted in a father's mind: I have lost my son. The Erik I knew is gone and will never return. He and I will never be the same.

Our impaired son had landed in an environment quite dissimilar from that which he had known just a short time earlier. I call disability a "kingdom" because it is an underclass as much as it is a place. All who enter the kingdom bear marks that set them apart from those without disabilities and even from their previous selves. Through standardized protocols, rehabilitation aimed to restore as much capability as possible in three months and to give an admittedly altered sense of purpose to Erik. Achieving this aim, however, was not easy given that we could not distinguish agitation caused by the brain injury from irritability provoked by awaking in a strange place with profoundly limited awareness and abilities. In our experience even the psychologists and social workers, who might have helped most in the momentous spiritual tasks of assimilating loss and of self-redefinition, focused principally on diagnostics and on preventing the psychological denial of disability. Little appreciation for the history of injury or of the patient prior to injury was readily expressed.

In contrast to the medical narrative, which was constructed largely out of sight and out of our reach, the rehabilitation narrative was more visible and available. Therapists functioned more like a dramatic cast of characters, often playing off the work of one another, than as individual narrators. Just as in the medical world, our role in the rehabilitation world had to be negotiated. Typically, local parents of patients in rehab visited in the evenings and took their family member home on weekends whenever possible. Occasionally parents would attend therapy sessions. Though the Dupont professionals also initially encouraged us to leave Erik in their care and to resume our daily lives back in our hometown, when they observed our willingness to extend the stimulation and exercises that they did with Erik in their formal sessions into other hours of the day, most of them accepted our involvement.

As a dramatic enactment of a story requires—each actor listening for cues, responding and supporting the other actors in the performances— the organization of the rehabilitation environment was more interactive and democratic than hierarchical and authoritarian. To be sure, we witnessed evidences of hierarchical privilege, enjoyed especially by those with medical degrees; however, a team approach to treatment generally equalized the participation of each therapist, and various kinds of interventions occurred simultaneously. There seemed to be far more flexibility of schedule in the Dupont rehabilitation setting. The medical staff sometimes worked around therapy schedules, and therapy sessions occasionally shifted to alternative times to accommodate a necessary medical procedure. In sum, to return to the image of the hammock that continued to swing in my imagination, the hammock was now being plaited through the collaborative activities that contributed to restoring and re-storying Erik's life.

Though Erik began to receive speech, physical, and occupational therapies from the day of his arrival, each of these therapies was directed by Erik's body-brain. In the rehabilitation environment we discovered more about the collaboration of the sensory and motor systems and the ways these are bound up with perception, psychology, and cognition. We learned experientially what M. Merleau-Ponty describes theoretically: "There is no physiological definition of sensation, and more generally there is no physiological psychology which is autonomous, because the physiological event itself obeys biological and psychological laws."[1] David Abram enlarges the investigation of the participatory nature of perception from human beings to the whole sensuous earth in his magical and wise *The Spell of the Sensuous*.[2] As I read Abram's work a dozen years after witnessing the reawakening of Erik's perceptions and their participatory character, my early intuition that our interaction with Erik and the communication going on within his own body-brain were part of a vast animated web of life force was profoundly confirmed.

The first abilities that each therapy addressed were rudimentary ones, beginning, as it were, in the brain stem. For the speech therapist, oral movements that would assist swallowing were critical. For the medical team, concern for Erik's unrestricted breathing was paramount. They began to assess the condition of the trachea and esophagus and to determine when the solid tube might be exchanged for a fenestrated one and when the tube might be removed altogether. The nursing staff initiated their carefully developed bowel training program, which was important not only as Erik moved from liquid and soft diets to solid foods but also for his later independence and self-care. The early weeks of physical therapy activity focused on gross motor movements—largely walking and balance, which would allow him to leave his wheelchair and to walk unsupported—and on ways of protecting him from his uncoordinated movements, such as his persistent efforts to stand upright in bed at all hours of the day or night during the early weeks.

Even though I can describe this range of early rehabilitative interventions in the space of one paragraph, each task represented a series of patient repetitions and sometimes complex and confusing negotiations. For example, after Erik's tongue relearned to move food from the front of the mouth to the back for swallowing without choking, Erik still could not pick up utensils, put food on them, or take the food to his mouth. He opened his mouth whenever we took food to it but was completely passive toward the tray in front of him. Over the course of two to three weeks the speech therapist and we worked to get him to indicate with his eyes when he wanted more food and which food he preferred. This was a time-consuming process, for often he didn't understand what we were asking him to do. Each meal was a practice in re-narrating his ability to relate his body's needs to resources outside his being that could supply those needs. With his tray of food before him we asked, Would you like? Do you want? If you want, can you show me with your eyes? Then we would wait, sometimes going over the questions two or three times and pointing to the various choices with a fork or spoon. Gradually, though inconsistently, some connection seemed to occur, and he would slowly move his eyes to a particular food.

The first goal of the bowel training program in any rehabilitation program is simply to keep the patient's digestive and elimination systems functioning well, but the values of regularity and eventual self-care lay embedded within it. Initially all responsibility in Erik's bowel training program was assumed by the staff, who administered the medications at night that would stimulate elimination in the morning. The staff aroused patients from their sleep to put them on the toilet or cleaned the beds when they did not get to the toilets in time. Because we stayed with Erik through the nights and were attuned to the nuances of his erratic rhythms, I began to sense, as I had when he was initially being toilet trained, when he needed to relieve himself. As we picked up these physical cues from him we expanded his narrative, as it were. We could respond promptly and communicate with Erik what we had detected from his body. By so doing we became part of a feedback loop between his disorganized interior and the external world. Feelings of satisfaction, both physical and psychological, could be experienced and reinforced through the simple description of the process in which we were engaged. Gradually, over many weeks, Erik became aware enough to resume responsibility for his own toileting.

Such early collaborative and intensive rehabilitation efforts filled us with renewed purpose and hope. Not only did we see evidence of small changes in Erik but also we could give visible direction to our concern for our son by learning the therapy routines ourselves and working with

him. Our rising sense of purpose, however, was deflated one late July
evening when the medical director and the neurologist brought the results of a new CT scan to discuss with us. As Erik's nurse readied him
for bed, we met in a nearby conference room, where we saw yet another
picture of Erik's brain and the blotchy patches indicating scarring.
Whereas when we had asked at the acute care hospital about the long-
term prognosis, we had received evasive responses, the neurologist and
medical director took the question head-on, though they hedged cau-
tiously. Both predicted that he might be able to finish high school if he
didn't plateau before regaining full consciousness, which seemed unlikely at the present moment. Any advanced learning beyond high
school would be highly unlikely in the best of outcomes, they thought.
He could perhaps complete high school because of what he already had
stored in the brain, but the ability to process new learning was severely
compromised by damage to the frontal lobes. The prevailing neuroscientific assumption was that damaged brain cells could not regenerate,
so though they left the door open a crack for some inexplicable "mira-
cle," both professionals felt fairly confident that their prognosis was a
responsible one. I also believe that they thought we as parents needed to
face and begin to accept this reality sooner rather than later.

As we returned to Erik's room with the weight of realization seared
on our hearts, I felt trapped between the desire to collapse in despair and
exhaustion and the determination not to give up. Although the tension
between grief and hope was familiar to us, we had just been handed an
interpretation of our son's condition that asked us to abandon all our assumptions about him and required us to imagine an entirely different
life story and set of goals for him that would affect all the rest of us in
the family. In Erik's room the nurse on duty intuited that we were
wrestling with dashed dreams and the shattered narrative of our son's
life. The interpretation we had just heard carried the sound of divine
predestination within it. It was like having someone reveal the ending
of a gripping novel when one is engrossed in the details and mystery.
Even though we knew we wanted to do all we could to assist Erik, no

matter what the outcome, how could we accept the loss of our former son and our aspirations as parents? Acceptance was virtually impossible at that moment, but we learned at that July evening conference that it was not helpful to tie our daily actions to past or future long-term goals. Instead we began to be more honest about wobbling between the disintegration of our son's identity and our family framework, on the one hand, and our persistent search to make meaning out of the fortuitous, on the other.

Our vulnerability, which the summer evening conversation had deepened, was intensified a few days later with the visit of three of Erik's high school friends. When they arrived I tried to describe what they should expect when they saw Erik, and I invited them to interact as fully and normally with him as possible, despite his lack of response. The poignant contrast between the integrated, promising lives that each of them was still enjoying and Erik's chaos was almost unbearable. They came hesitantly but respectfully, bearing gifts: a shirt wrapped tidily in sunflower gold paper and a wide, deep purple ribbon, several packages of Toblerone chocolate, and a small, plastic aquarium suitcase containing two energetic goldfish. I ached to see my son in his friends' tanned and agile bodies. How could I love them and resent their gracefully integrated mind-bodies? The question hurt too much, so I quickly climbed on my thread and moved toward the ceiling to get a "larger," more tolerant view and to flee from the depths of loss. Though I did not wish Erik's circumstances on anyone else, I resisted strenuously the fact that our son would be unable to reengage with his friends in the way he had before the accident. Indeed, if the predictions we had heard just days before were accurate, he would never return to the college preparatory classes at Princeton Day School. Throughout the remainder of the summer at Dupont, the impact of the medical director's and the neurologist's prognosis was lightened by almost weekly visits from a couple of Erik's teachers and small groups of friends. Our efforts to give meaning to the disintegration of our son's life were gradually overshadowed by the ordinary, regular rehabilitation necessities that ordered our days. And so we clung to those.

Within a day or two of the pessimistic prognosis the pulmonary physician replaced the solid trach tube with a fenestrated one. Now we could hear Erik's voice again in soft cries and whimpers. To hear the voice of our child after six weeks of absolute silence lifted our dejected spirits enormously. First, hearing the sounds relieved our fear that the vocal cords might have been damaged from the surgical procedure or the insertion of the various tubes early in his hospitalization. Our encouragement was tempered by the doctor, who, while exchanging the tubes, discovered that quite a lot of scar tissue had formed around the tube, which could present problems later when he tried to remove the tube altogether. Second, despite this anxiety-producing caution, and even though we could only speculate about and interpret the "meaning" of his sounds through our frame of reference, I did feel that another channel of potential communication had been reopened for us.

Throughout the rehabilitation process Erik fluctuated between agitation and heightening awareness. During the first three weeks at Dupont his agitation seemed most severe at night, often waking him as if with an adrenaline rush that awkwardly but strongly lifted him to his knees and quickly to his feet on his hospital bed. Most efforts to calm him, like quiet, reassuring talk, gentle but firm physical pressure to seat him, or familiar classical music—John Williams on guitar, the Bach Brandenburg concertos, Mozart or Brahms symphonies played softly on his portable tape recorder—failed. Wanting as much as possible to take our cues from Erik's own body-brain, Robert concluded that letting him walk during these agitated states rather than physically restraining him in his bed, which was typical hospital protocol in such extreme cases, would most effectively relieve the agitation. We negotiated with the night staff to walk with Erik around the halls each night until the agitation dissipated. Sometimes Erik and Robert walked the empty corridors repeatedly throughout the night. Then Erik returned to bed and usually restful sleep.

Erik's nighttime walks now bring to mind Charles Dickens's description of his own experiment with night walking to relieve "a temporary inability to sleep, referable to a distressing impression." Although the purpose of Dickens's walks, as he narrates them in "Night Walks," was to get through the night, he found that houselessness "brought [him] into sympathetic relations with people who have no other object every night in the year." Traveling through London to Newgate or along the Old Kent road or to a tavern or to Billingsgate, Old Bailey, and Bethlehem Hospital, Dickens wonders, "Are not the sane and the insane equal at night as the sane lie a-dreaming? Are not all of us outside this hospital, who dream, more or less in the condition of those inside it, every night of our lives?"[3] Walking the silent hospital corridors at night, passing dark therapy rooms that during the day resounded with activity and struggle, talking quietly to our son, who, although still in his familiar body, seemed houseless in mind and spirit and needful of some abiding place and connections, I longed to know what sights he must be seeing, imagining, fearing. What electrical physical signals were being rerouted in the brain, what passageways slightly unclogged or swept by the movement of his torso and limbs? Was he moving in thick fog, totally disoriented from any horizon? Was he having inner visions or meeting memory fragments as we passed along in silence? By walking with him were we bringing him closer to home? And what would home mean?

Medical and rehabilitation concerns that such activity in the middle of the night might make Erik groggy for therapies were occasionally borne out, for Erik did sometimes seem more sleepy the day immediately following his nighttime walks. Over many weeks, however, we detected a subtle pattern of change in Erik's level of awareness two or three days following these agitated walkabouts. It seemed to us as if something in his disheveled brain "sorted" itself out slightly during these periods of extreme agitation and the body's physical response through movement, and the coma lightened yet another degree. Walking seemed to connect his brain with his muscles through motor activity and thereby connect both with his conscious mind.

The frequency of these night periods of agitation gradually diminished over the space of a month, although Erik could experience periods of volatile emotional outburst at almost any time when he felt frustrated. In many ways Erik exhibited behaviors like those of a caged animal. Being trapped inside a body with diminished abilities that he did not recognize as his own, despite compromised self-awareness, and lacking language, compounded the agitation. Every probing investigation, such as CT scans that required him to be inserted into a tubelike tunnel or examinations of his trachea with a scope for scar tissue, seemed threatening and invasive to Erik, thereby heightening his sense of entrapment and confusion.

When in early August the doctors finally decided it was time to remove the tube from his trachea, they first plugged the hole for several hours at a time to see how his breathing would be affected. When it was clear that he could breathe independently, it took two surgical procedures a week apart—in addition to one that had to be aborted because the anaesthetic was administered too long before the actual procedure—to free the fenestrated tube from the rapidly forming, prolific scar tissue. The first procedure made an incision to remove scar tissue. The second removed the tube and closed the hole. Even after the tube was removed the doctor had to monitor the trachea closely to ensure that scar tissue would not grow back in such a way that it would shut off the air passage.

The removal of the trach tube returned the potential for language to Erik. Would he speak? we wondered as we waited anxiously through the surgeries. *Could* he speak? He did not speak right after the tube was removed. We were sad but not hopeless. When Robert put him to bed later that first night without the trach tube, he was talking to him as he always did and told Erik matter-of-factly to lie down. Suddenly Erik began to repeat a sound like *lie, lie, lie* over and over. But he didn't speak. The next morning Robert assisted him while getting up, talking to him as usual. He again told Erik his own name, that he had had an accident, and that he was his dad. Suddenly Erik repeated "Dad" several times. Robert was overjoyed, for this was a moment of great hope. "Erik," Robert said, "Do you know me? Do you know I'm your dad?" Erik kept saying "Dad, Dad, Dad" over and over, as if he wanted to hear it or liked the sound of it himself. To explore whether this was real or some accidental series of sounds, Robert asked, "Erik, can you say 'Mom'? She will be here soon." Erik said "Mom, Mom, Mom." Robert knew this was real, mindful communication. He jumped up and down, hugged Erik in his wheelchair in the bathroom, exclaiming, "This is wonderful beyond my wildest dreams. You are talking to me. Thank God, we can have a life together again." By the time I arrived at the hospital later that morning Erik was repetitively saying "Mom," "Dad," and "Sonia." The presence of language would change the orientation of all his therapies, the level of his coma, and the nature of his agitation. His first speech was imitative, just as it had been when he was an infant learning language.

The ability to speak dramatically lightened Erik's coma, revealing how dependent what we consider selfhood is on consciousness and language. We were elated to hear our son speak, even if only single, repeated words. I thought, despite what I had felt just two weeks earlier, that even if Erik's condition did not improve further I would be grateful simply that we could communicate, however rudimentarily. Somehow the restored capacity to produce sound brought him back into communication with a universe vibrant with sounds and confirmed our own dependence on sound for relationship and identity.

Because the trach tube was removed on a Friday afternoon we had the weekend to investigate and experiment with Erik's language. Instinctively I began to combine some of the physical activities that we did with him when he wasn't in formal therapies with his new vocal-verbal ability. Tossing a soccer ball had become a favorite free-time activity. As we tossed the ball back and forth between us I began to recite nursery rhymes in rhythm to our tossing. After a few full rhymes I stopped after a phrase: "Hickory, dickory ———." I waited to see if Erik would supply the missing word. At first I repeated the phrase and waited, and then Erik supplied "dock." I continued, "The mouse ran up the ———." My wait this time was much shorter as he caught on and offered "clock." For the next ten to fifteen minutes we rhythmically ran through our old repertoire of childhood rhymes. If anyone had told me three months earlier that I would be exhilarated by learning that our sixteen-year-old son, who a few months earlier had loved the challenges of physics and calculus, could retrieve words from nursery rhymes, I would have believed that person mad.

Sonia had been preparing a photograph album for Erik to help him piece his life story back together. She selected photos from his infancy and childhood, of relatives, of treasured Christmases and birthday parties and labeled each one carefully. On the weekend that Erik was free of the trach tube she had the album ready and brought it proudly to him at the hospital. Instead of accepting this helpful gesture of love, Erik at first simply shut the book and his eyes when Sonia tried to leaf through it with him. Was it too much unrecognizable detail or possibly too much confusingly recognizable experience that produced this pain? This was the first of many subsequent times Sonia would attempt to reach and to reclaim a relationship with a brother she had known and admired. We noted her visible disappointment, affirmed the significance of her gift, and predicted that his response would change, as indeed it did by the end of that day, when he focused for a few minutes on the book and even named a few relatives.

With so much of our attention riveted to the rehabilitation of Erik, what had regrettably dropped from our view was the casualty of our daughter's self-identity inflicted by her older brother's losses. As parents we had life narratives that preexisted our children's entry into our stories. We had a reservoir of experience, knowledge, and faith—however inadequate they were to these challenges—on which to draw. For Sonia, when Erik's life as she had known it was ripped from her, her own life, never lived without him, seemed set adrift.

At about the same time that the trach tube was removed we observed a fleeting but very disturbing phenomenon in Erik's facial expression. Occasionally replacing the blank, fixed gaze was a one-sided smile that looked sneering and malevolent. The cause of this expression was never explained. Later, upon reading Antonio Damasio's research on the ways emotions and bodily sensations influence conscious awareness, and how injuries to the frontal cortex subsequently may affect the capacity for moral decision making, I wondered fleetingly if the sneer suggested a temporary impairment to Erik's ability to make moral distinctions.[4] We knew that he had sustained injury to the frontal cortex, which lies just behind the eye sockets and near the bridge of the nose. The normal inhibitions that people learn were not present. Although it was initially disturbing, Robert and I wanted intuitively to accept the sneer and welcome it because it represented an advance over a vacant face. It suggested a step toward expressing emotion and providing texture to life. We sought to welcome all expressions of feeling and color, believing that a "return" to life needed to precede the refinement of it. Fortunately the sneering expression gradually disappeared as consciousness and his capacity for language increased.

Observing Erik's use of language shortly after the trach tube had been removed, I realized that language might be to cognition as walking was to consciousness. Both walking and speaking seemed to possess organizing potential and connective possibilities for the brain. Walking appeared to soothe Erik's disordered brain, manifested as physical agitation; the movement in space seemed to connect him to himself, the comatose state moving toward awakening. Erik's initial speaking was much like repetitive walking, for it was imitative (characterized as echolalia) and perseverative. Whereas on their nighttime walks Erik and Robert might go round and round the same hallways, in speaking Erik picked up a word or phrase in a conversation and repeated it again and again and again. This behavior was easy to identify when Erik imitated words from our conversations with him, but the significance of the echolalia to his relationship with others and the world outside his head or room became clear when I walked with him in the hallway and in the hospital gardens soon after he could form speech sounds again. Until I caught on to what was taking place, I thought Erik was bizarrely uttering nonsensical groups of words. For example, we could be walking along a hallway when suddenly he might say, "it didn't have gas," or "call back at 11 o'clock," or "running into trouble." Where did these come from? I wondered. They seemed to come out of nowhere. Then one day I realized that these phrases often popped out of his mouth right after others, speaking to one another, had passed us in the hall. These phrases that seemed random were in fact picked up, radarlike, by Erik's brain and acute hearing, and he inserted them randomly into our conversation. I interpreted this as his way of experimentally navigating in a world that must have seemed dreamlike.

Instead of letting this primitive language attempt dangle in the air unacknowledged, when I realized what was occurring I asked him if he had heard those people whom we had passed saying the particular phrase he had just uttered. At first he did not respond, for imitative speech is not deliberate and, in Erik's case at this time, not in full consciousness. I tried to weave his random phrase into our conversation by suggesting what those people we had just passed might have been discussing when they spoke the phrase he had repeated. After a few efforts to bind his words into our communication and to insinuate, through his echoed words, a relationship with people in the surrounding space, he responded affirmatively to my question about whether he was repeating what he had just heard. Within a relatively short time most of the echolalia ceased, encouraged by his rising consciousness and perhaps by our attempts to incorporate his capacity to speak purposelessly into a narrative that over time aroused him to the presence of others and the ways language constructs relationships. When he was tired or under stress of any sort, the echolalia would resume.

Our enthusiasm for Erik's returning language capacity challenged our own control and propriety patterns, although such challenges did not daunt our encouragement of his attempts at self-expression. We were not too surprised to hear a few words of profanity coming from his mouth when he was agitated or expressing himself with repeated words, for they seemed as random as most of his other words. But one evening as we walked outside on the hospital grounds amidst the summer sounds of birds and crickets settling in the twilight, Erik's mouth became a virtual fountain of perseverative profanity. As we passed other patients and their families or visitors approaching the hospital, Erik let loose a barrage of profane expletives, over and over. He was not visibly agitated but seemed simply to be exercising his language ability. What a bind for parents who had tried to teach their children to be polite to friends and strangers and had discouraged cursing! We were grateful for any emotional and verbal expression, however, so we calmly smiled at passersby as our son peppered the air with his "bad" language. At that moment not only were my own standards of propriety called into question, for I was not about to tell my son who had been stone silent for six weeks to shush, but also I realized that no language is, in and of itself, bad; only our thinking makes it so.

Little incidents, easily ignored by most people, became significant in our imaginations. For example, one evening as he prepared Erik for bed Robert was summarizing the activities of his day. Erik picked out a few words here and there from Robert's chronicle of the day's events, saying them over and over again. Suddenly from the hallway came peals of laughter. Erik stopped his mindless repetition and said "laughter," illustrating some ability to distinguish other sounds outside himself from those he had been imitating and a capacity for abstraction: he had generalized laughing voices into the concept of laughter. Although this was, to be sure, a crude illustration of abstract thinking or association, I interpreted it as a harbinger of future developments. As we experimented with Erik's reacquisition of language, I felt like a child myself, trying to guess at meaning or to link his loose words to objects. Indeed, it seemed as if we were all reacquiring language ability. Erik was trying to locate lost words and we were guessing, smiling, pointing, and affixing names to objects for him. I recalled a passage from Augustine, describing his own transition from infancy to childhood, in which he depicts the linguistic and relational foundation of every self and of the will.

> When they [my elders] named any thing, and as they spoke turned towards it, I saw and remembered that they called what they would point out by the name they uttered. And that they meant this thing and no other was plain from the motion of their body, the natural language, as it were, of all [people], expressed by the countenances, glances of the eye, gestures of the limbs, and tones of the voice, indicating the affections of the mind, as it pursues, possesses, rejects, or shuns. And thus by constantly hearing words, as they occurred in various sentences, I collected gradually for what they stood; and having broken in my mouth to these signs, I thereby gave utterance to my will.[5]

With the return of language capability two important challenges became clearly visible and both necessary and possible to address. First, the reacquisition of language turned all Erik's therapies in a more cognitive direction. Second, the reality of social maladaptation associated with brain injury became obvious. After Erik had rudimentary language ability each therapist worked at communicating with Erik through conversation; they no longer needed to assume answers for him or ask him to point with eyes or fingers. Only a few days after Erik began speaking we put a sign in his room with his name on it. When he read "Erik Jo," leaving off the "hansen," we happily supplied the last two syllables. Quickly he confirmed his ability to read, as he had his speaking, by reading parts of signs he saw around the hospital or in his therapy rooms or by selecting a word or two from therapy directions that were printed.

As the speech therapist intensified her cognitive work with Erik she observed two important tendencies in his language behavior: he seemed better able to attach words to feelings than to objects or cognitive tasks, and he seemed to depend more on auditory than on visual perception for tackling cognitive tasks, for he performed assigned tasks better

when the therapist spoke the instructions aloud or he read them labori-
ously out loud himself. Because we had not previously known whether
our son was more an auditory than a visual learner or whether his preference for processing information and experiences was through feeling
more than thinking, neither we nor the therapist could determine the
extent to which the tendencies he now exhibited were consequences of
his injury. Several months later, however, a neuropsychologist asked to
see some of Erik's essays and a research paper that he had written for
school assignments prior to the accident. From a close examination of
his use of language in those written compositions the neuropsychologist
concluded that Erik relied more heavily on feelings as he interacted with
his environment. An awareness of this tendency to rely on feeling as the
first avenue for interpreting experiences and sense impressions, and the
cognitive implications of this mode of processing, would become increasingly important for Erik's rehabilitation in the subsequent months
and years.

The return of language brought the clinical psychologist more directly
into Erik's rehabilitation schedule. Erik began to meet at least once or
twice a week with Dr. Adams for cognitive and psychological assessment.
After their first session together Dr. Adams reported that Erik seemed
to have good short-term memory and recommended that we capitalize
on that. He made no judgment or predictions about his long-term
memory or his retention capability. The sessions varied, depending on
Erik's attention span, how rested he was, and other indeterminable factors that supported or interrupted his engagement with such tasks as putting shapes in their proper space on a board or counting backward or
forward by sevens or tens. Over the remaining six weeks at Dupont, Dr.
Adams administered a battery of psychological and intelligence tests to
assess Erik's post-accident abilities. At the conclusion of one of Erik's sessions, Dr. Adams casually mentioned the likelihood that Erik would
need to be placed in a special education classroom when it was possible
for him to return to school. The cognitive and emotional deficits with
which he would have to contend would make a regular classroom ex-

ceedingly difficult, he said. This prediction registered deeply in my being, reminding me again of the news we'd received from the medical
director and neurologist a few weeks earlier, although I was not prepared
to respond to it or question it at that moment. When I later reported this
brief exchange to Robert we once again felt caught between our aspirations for the best possible outcome for our son and the rehabilitation staff
members' interpretations of realistic probabilities. Their narrative was
not and could not be ours.

In addition to receiving cognitive therapy with the speech therapist
and psychologist, Erik began to spend more time in the classroom containing computers. Because Erik had loved computer activities before
his injury and had enjoyed creating graphics programs alone and with
some of his friends, we expected that the opportunity to work on the
computer would arouse his interest. To be sure, over many weeks and
months that previous interest seemed to return, but to a greatly diminished degree. Initially, however, Erik sat blankly before the key-
board and screen; he had to be coached step-by-step to reengage with the
computer, and at first he seemed not to recognize the connection between what he did with his hands and what appeared on the screen.
Gradually, with persistent direction by the educational specialist, Erik
could do simple computer exercises to refine spatial organization skills,
to increase his attention span, to strengthen his memory. Performing
these computer exercises was tedious, and often his frustration erupted
in random and belligerent moving of the joy stick or pushing away from
the computer altogether.

The heightened attention to Erik's cognitive capacities in all his therapies revealed how practical and object-tied most rehabilitation therapies are. For example, the primary goal in occupational therapy was to
help Erik become functional and independent in basic self-care. With
the return of language and his ability to read individual words, the focus of occupational therapy evolved from tasks that required eye-hand
coordination, memory skills, and management of personal care activities like dressing or washing to include those requiring more cognitive

involvement such as locating states or countries on a map or looking up names and phone numbers in a telephone directory. Eventually he was challenged to read a recipe and follow simple directions for making pizza.

In addition to shifting attention to Erik's cognitive functioning, the return of language produced a social challenge. Just as cognitive and physical abilities are confounded by brain injury, so too are the affective dimensions of human personality on which selfhood and all social interactions depend. As Erik's level of consciousness increased and he resumed speaking, his words were often socially inappropriate. Although uttering streaks of profanity in public spaces as one emerges from coma might not strictly speaking be regarded as socially inappropriate behavior, if such expressions become standard parts of one's efforts to talk to others or to grab attention, they do become inappropriate. Diminished cognitive capacities, limited vocabulary, and a strong desire for relationship, combined with the frustration that accompanies emotional confusion or physical disabilities, often result in bizarre behaviors among those with acquired brain injuries. Any accidental, socially inappropriate action that produces a strong response of laughter or criticism may be repeated for the attention it produces. Sexually suggestive language and behavior commonly occur among the brain injured, especially young males. Erik was no exception. One day as I walked a little distance behind Erik and Robert, I noticed Erik's Bermuda shorts gradually slipping down over his hips. I began to laugh as I caught up with them, thinking that the pants were falling because of Erik's weight loss and that both males were oblivious to the situation. When I reached them and informed them that Erik's pants were dropping I realized that Erik seemed to enjoy my laughter and that he may have initiated the slippage by pushing his hands strongly down into the pockets. This behavior had to be interrupted several more times without drawing unusual attention to it. Sexual innuendo or sexualized comments made toward others also often elicit peals of laughter from those who do not recognize that the brain injured are trying to renegotiate social relationships. The challenge family members and others who work with the brain injured face is to figure out how to interrupt without moral condemnation or reinforcement of the inappropriate behavior.

Several conclusions became clear to us as we worked with Erik on socially appropriate behaviors over the weeks and months and, with increasing subtlety, over the years. We did not want to ignore or belittle Erik's personhood as we tried not to call undue attention to any inappropriate action. We often tried to redirect the conversation or supply alternative language as we acknowledged what seemed to be underlying or precipitating feelings that yielded a less than socially acceptable reaction. We also made every effort to be consistent in our responses to repeated inappropriate behaviors so as not to confuse Erik further with fluctuating responses. Above all, despite our own embarrassment or even occasional anger at the outburst of any uncouth or crude behavior, we tried to look beneath such words or actions for a fuller appreciation of our son, who was struggling to reorient his self within his own psyche and in his social relations. This was quite possible for us to do because at every point we could remember: although flawed or imperfect, this behavior is much better than death or coma.

All the repetitive activities that ordered Erik's days and nights at the Dupont Children's Hospital often seemed like an endlessly circling series of mediative and interpretive tasks necessary for reclothing what we so casually call the self. Each day that Erik practiced running or maintaining his balance, lifted weights on pulleys, or tried to catch and throw a ball, he was bridging the chasm between his physical deficits and his former physical agility. In speech and occupational therapies his relearning of basic cognitive, language, and self-care skills mediated between a confused, isolated mental state and the complex interactions required in social community.

Throughout his inpatient rehabilitation Erik often said, "Get me out of this nightmare." Especially in the dark of night, as he was preparing for bed, or when he awakened in the night to go to the bathroom he said, "Am I dead? Wake me up. I feel like I'm in a nightmare." One

particular evening he said, "A great accident has left me brainless."
When I said, "Not brainless," he revised his comment: "Left me smart-
less." During this time Erik angrily resisted his occupational therapist—
accidentally calling her by the name of an aunt he experienced as
domineering—and some of the activities directed by the speech therapist. Entangled in his night dreams and his statements of living in a
nightmare were aggressive remarks, peppered with profanity, about a
cousin with learning disabilities and references to a deceased great aunt
who experienced severe dementia in the last years of her life.

None of the rehabilitation therapies, all directed toward behavioral
change, addressed these psychic issues, which were arising from the injured brain and the unconscious. Upon visiting Erik in August, our long-
time friend and Jungian psychoanalyst James Hollis suggested that Erik
was working in the unconscious to piece his life back together in reality. He explained that whereas nightmares in adults usually signal unresolved issues, in a child they indicate that something traumatic has occurred. Jim speculated that Erik's references to his great aunt whose
mind became confused and to his cousin with learning difficulties symbolized what he feared in himself. Ideally Erik should have received
metaphoric therapy along with behavioral therapy. In conversations with
the speech therapist about Erik's dream references, I asked how we might
best explore these with him. She suggested we get a referral to a child
psychologist who worked with dreams. Preliminary explorations about
such a referral revealed two things. Brain injured patients are not considered viable clients for such therapy because their cognitive abilities
are in flux and unreliable and their attention spans are relatively short.
More disturbingly, the medical community and insurance companies
alike operate with the bias that dual diagnoses do not exist. Because
brain injury carries a neurological diagnosis, the psychological reactions
to it are considered a separate diagnosis and are generally left unaddressed in the rehabilitation world. Nevertheless, we continued to respect Erik's symbolic life, to allow him to express the fears that he ex-

perienced in his dreams or that he expressed during waking activities, and to ask him questions that might help him piece his shattered self-story back together.

Although we had no professional verification of the nature of dream activity in the brain injured or even guidance about how to investigate the dream world, which is so dependent on image and emotion, we were convinced on the basis of anecdotal evidence that something valuable was occurring beneath the surface of activities that were designed to reorganize Erik's behaviors and awareness, and that his daily regimen of therapies would help him reshape the manifest level of his personal narrative. But largely hidden from view, though erupting occasionally and dismissed as agitation, disorientation, or bizarre behavior, there was a latent dimension of struggle to re-narrate his life.

For example, a few days after Erik began to "speak" words, while he and Robert were returning from a physical therapy session, he suddenly, without any external provocation, began to scream loudly and with chilling emotion, "Can you see? Can you see? Can you see?" When Robert asked, "Can I see what?" Erik continued to shout the same phrase. After Robert asked a second time what Erik wanted him to see, he said "the *contilental*." Robert was stunned by this word, for the car in which Erik had been riding had been hit by a Lincoln Continental. We had never told him, nor to our knowledge had anyone else, that he had been hit by such a vehicle. Robert quickly tried to ask him some questions about what he could see, but by then the agitated "vision" had passed and Erik became more placid and unresponsive. For perhaps half a minute Erik had a window of consciousness open to what must have been the final moment of his former life, when he saw a Lincoln Continental bearing down on him.

Several times, either as he was settling into bed or upon waking from an apparent dream, Erik said, "I almost died, I almost died." Attempting to invite further expression, we asked him how that felt. All he ever said was "It was scary." He frequently reported dreams that included friends from earlier years in his life, references to animal and human sexuality, comments about a great aunt and great uncle who are deceased, and identification of himself with his cousin. On one occasion he reported that he had "electricity dust" in his eyes.

As Erik carried out the most arduous internal mediative challenges, Robert and I mediated between family and friends and Erik and sometimes between Erik and the hospital staff. Our task was to interpret Erik's condition or developments in his rehabilitation. Often we needed to be friendly yet firm advocates on his behalf. When I wrote letters to his school class before they spread out for summer vacations or to update extended family or our religious community on his status, I rigorously resisted labels that fixed his condition. Although others might say that I was living in some denial, I refused to describe Erik as brain damaged, always preferring to speak about the injuries to the brain and making space for changes that no one could adequately foresee. Those relatives and friends who came to visit Erik at Dupont without any information about traumatic brain injury were shocked at the profound changes in him, despite our informing them beforehand. We sometimes found ourselves standing between their horror and fear and our own gratitude that he had come so far. Their presence was a reminder of how vastly we as parents had been altered by this experience.

One of the most challenging mediative tasks to be carried out with family and friends as well as rehabilitation and medical professionals was learning how to express ideas or interests on behalf of our child that ran sharply counter to the preferences, directives, or even expertise of others. For example, family members or friends who came to visit with their own prominent needs for attention, care, or reassurance, or with a desire to advise, had to be helped to understand that Erik's energy was quite limited, as was that of those who worked with him daily. Those who offered their concern through anxious exclamations or by insisting, for example, on particular forms of prayer did not contribute to a healing environment. Nor did those who uncomfortably avoided interaction with Erik. Indeed, we discovered that feelings of tension or unresolved

conflicts between people registered visibly in Erik's body and in his behavior, just as they did within our own. Indeed, Robert and I struggled
between us to relinquish those things we could not control, such as Erik's
long-term outcome, as we simultaneously gave the fullest attention to
caring about and for him. To learn "to care and not to care,"[6] to mediate between vigorous interventions and stillness, was our daily challenge.

We were fortunate that, for the most part, our parents, brothers and
sister, their families, and our friends were able and willing to enter this
unraveled world of brain injury and learn about it with us, even by telephone across a thousand miles. When Erik's uncle and younger cousins
came 700 miles to visit and to return Sonia from her month-long vacation with grandparents and aunts and uncles in the Midwest, Erik recognized them. They all greeted him with total acceptance and affection,
quickly entering into his therapy exercises or making up games in
which Erik in his groggy state could participate.

Toward the end of the summer the rehabilitation staff suggested that
we prepare Erik for a weekend home visit by first taking him for a short
outing within Wilmington. Now we would have to mediate between the
security of the rehabilitation hospital and the fast-paced, sound-saturated
impersonality of the public world as we conveyed our vulnerable son between the two. We could not predict Erik's reactions to riding in a car
again after two months; we did not know what impressions of the accident might be imprinted in his psyche and how being in a car and in
traffic might stimulate his memory. We prepared him ahead of time for
the outing, trying to elicit from him a suggestion of where he might like
to go. He had no recommendation but seemed content with the idea that
we go to McDonald's for a shake. For Sonia and us this was a momentous, if anxious, occasion; Erik's reaction was quite flat. As we narrated
every step of this small journey, he complied agreeably to being belted
into the car, to having me sit next to him in the back seat, and to riding
almost glassy-eyed through traffic and past summer gardens. Only the
speed with which he drank his shake conveyed any enthusiasm. Before
returning to Dupont we stopped to visit the Hoovers, the couple in whose

home the three of us had been staying when we weren't at the hospital. With them Erik became more alert and engaged, confirming again the interdependent, interactive character of selfhood. We returned to Dupont satisfied with our first outing, but ready to let down our guard in the protection and care of now familiar surroundings.

Preparing for our first home visit the following weekend required more profound mediations than I anticipated. To return to the house we had left three months earlier filled each of us with anxiety and pain that we exhibited in individual ways. Of the four of us, Erik was least aware of, and hence less overtly troubled by, the impending return home. Sonia, who had been wishing and praying all summer that things would just get back to normal, seemed pleased that enough progress had occurred for Erik to go home, although underneath her cheerful demeanor lurked confusing thirteen-year-old emotions about how different, strange, and embarrassing this person, her brother, now was. Disagreements arose between Robert and me. I welcomed offers from friends to clean and prepare the house, but he preferred not to have such interventions into our private space and personal grief. Although I had wanted to rearrange Erik's room slightly, Robert insisted that we leave it exactly the way Erik had left it. This would be Robert's first overnight stay at home since the accident. He had refused to go home overnight as long as Erik could not. The accident continued to traumatize him and our family despite our efforts to accept that which we could not change. In any case, throughout the week we planned for all the contingencies we could imagine at home, gathered necessary equipment, medications, and supplies, attended Erik's regular therapies, and continued our ongoing narration of Erik's former life and present condition, of what he might remember of home and thereby somehow anticipate. Would anything seem familiar to him or arouse a more awakened response in him?

We had barely been home an hour on Friday evening—the last weekend in August—when a friend from the Friends Meeting, who had volunteered to take care of the children's dog, called and asked if he could bring Happy to the house to see Erik. John said he thought it might help

Erik to see his dog. Although we were reluctant and protective during this first sojourn home, we agreed. John was far wiser than we on this matter, for when he arrived and Erik and Happy met on the back deck, the moment of mutual recognition and affection was electric. Happy was totally beside himself with joy, giving licking kisses to Erik. Erik began to sob. This was the first expression of sadness, indeed of any connecting emotion, from Erik. All of us stood by with tears streaming unashamedly down our cheeks as Erik hugged and talked to Happy in his inflectionless voice, even offering him a piece of pizza. The encounter between Erik and Happy marked a significant shift in Erik's awareness. Even though he had been responding with fluctuating success to directives in all his therapies during the past several weeks, his responses had usually been lackluster and robotic. Following this emotional release and recognition, the remaining shreds of coma fell away.

As Erik's awareness of himself increased so did the occasions of irritation with others, especially Sonia. On Saturday of our second home visit Erik began expressing hostility toward her. Suggesting that I didn't think Sonia deserved his angry outburst, I asked whether he was upset because of the difficulties he faced as a result of the accident. He said yes and then asked me to tell him again about the accident. Whenever he asked for any kind of information or help we tried to provide it in a question and answer format that we thought might help him pull from memory or piece together information he already possessed. Although we had told him the accident story several times before, he had not retained any accurate details. As we sat talking about the accident in his bedroom, he looked at his book shelf and suddenly asked, "When does school start?" "September 10th," I replied. "What date is it today?" he asked. "August 31st," I said. And Erik began to cry. Although I really didn't need to ask why he was crying, I did, and he replied brokenly, through his sobs, "Because I won't be going to school." He walked to his shelf and pulled off his calculus book, sobbing deeply as he said, "Math was my best subject. I was good in math." We all cried together, holding one another. Soon Erik said, "Don't cry, Dad. Don't worry about me."

The pain of his realization settled more deeply upon us at home in the presence of reminders of his interests and abilities no longer viable at this time. At Dupont we happily encouraged Erik in his cognitive and educational therapies as he was relearning to write his name, to do simple addition and subtraction, to recite the multiplication tables, and to struggle through reading comprehension paragraphs, but here at home the discontinuity between his present capabilities and his earlier ones devastated us. Within the space of twenty-four hours the previous weekend the lingering veil of coma that had separated us from our son had finally lifted, and, stimulated through the release of emotion, Erik exhibited some primitive grasp of the threshold on which he now existed, a mysterious space between a former self and an unknown being who was under construction. I wondered how we could walk with him in the narrow, dark valley that divided the past from the future without giving up.

The successful home visits signaled the approaching conclusion of Erik's inpatient rehabilitation and our need to imagine and create ways to continue Erik's rehabilitation outside the protected environment of the Dupont Children's Hospital. As the medical and rehabilitation staffs, along with the social worker, suggested one more month for Erik at Dupont, they also recommended options for us to consider as we planned to return to the everyday world of busy schedules, professional responsibilities, rapid transit, and the restless pursuit of goals. The mediations that Robert and I had carried out with the Dupont staff from the time of our arrival were compounded as we anticipated release and as the various prognoses and interpretations of Erik's condition and needs became more complicated.

From the beginning of this journey with traumatic brain injury we found ourselves swinging between a scientific-instrumentalist approach to the injured human body that pervades Western medicine and a spiritual faith informed by our own Anabaptist-Pietist background and other religious traditions. From Anabaptist history we knew about persecution and suffering for one's faith and valued the Anabaptists' unwillingness to conform themselves to temporal values. Pietism instructed us in the immanence, as well as transcendence, of God's reality and in the possibility of continued, direct revelation. From Buddhism and Taoism we had come to appreciate balance, harmony, and the transformative power of meditation, as well as the presence of suffering in all life. Our responses to the challenges Erik faced were always shaped by both poles: the scientific-technical and the ineffable. Despite the practical, concrete goals of rehabilitation, our private interactions with Erik included regular meditation and prayer for him, especially as he slept at night.

The relevance and therapeutic potential of the meditative and imaginative approach to Erik's impairments was illustrated one evening as Robert helped Erik prepare for bed. The physical therapist had been addressing the lack of flexibility in Erik's feet and toes for several days. Unable to bend his toes, he clumped along flat-footedly when he walked. As Erik settled into bed and after their customary time of quiet prayer, Robert gently rubbed Erik's feet, slowly bending his toes back and forth. As he did this, he asked Erik to close his eyes and try to feel the movement in his toes and then to imagine his brain making connections that would move his toes for him. After several minutes of this, Robert stopped moving Erik's toes and asked Erik if he could move them by himself. They both sat there without speaking for what seemed a long time. Robert repeated the pattern again, and again asked Erik if he could move his toes on his own. Finally, just as Robert was about ready to give up for the night and pull the blankets up, Erik's toes moved slightly. Both father and son were elated, and for the next several days in the morning and evening they repeated this exercise patiently.

For the most part the Dupont staff respectfully ignored our meditation exercises with or on behalf of Erik, although on two or three occasions the medical director, neurologist, psychologist, and even the social worker urged us to face the reality of Erik's condition and go home more. As we prepared to leave the rehabilitation hospital and to plan for some kind of partial reentry into society, greater differences in interpretations of the "meaning" of Erik's changes arose sometimes between us and the staff, sometimes among therapists and the social worker. The underlying question was what was necessary and appropriate for Erik.

On this point the characteristics of the story enacted in the rehabilitation world stood out in bold relief against the personal interpretations and applications of that overarching narrative. During the three months that we had been at Dupont we began to understand the central themes and goals of the rehab narrative through the therapy protocols adapted for each patient. These protocols, developed from treating patients with injured spinal cords, individuals impaired by strokes, and people with gunshot or war wounds, had as their common goal the patient's basic functionality. Patients were re-clothed through the restoration of their abilities to negotiate with the objective world around them, which required them to create or to discover an "objective" view of themselves with their altered capacities in that world. When patients were able to manage these negotiations the rehabilitation narrative was considered largely finished.

While it appeared that Erik had recovered a simple biological consciousness, what Damasio calls *core consciousness* and defines as an organism's sense of itself at one moment and in one place, his *extended consciousness* remained underdeveloped and sometimes in apparent disarray.[7] Recognizing how far Erik was from his former capacity for engaging the complex multidimensional operations of the social world and pondering, from my earliest realization of what had happened to him, questions about the location of his self or the existence of some essence, I saw that these functionalist goals of rehabilitation did not adequately clothe Erik. They were undeniably important, but I knew dimly that we were only at the beginning of the long road we would travel with Erik, despite the standard presumption in 1985 that most of what a brain injured patient would be likely to recover could be expected in the first six months to one year. Those therapists and the psychologist who seemed most closely tied to the rehabilitation metanarrative counseled us to request placement of Erik in our public school system's special education program to meet his educational needs and then to supplement with in-home physical therapy. A few others, who perhaps understood better that many special education classrooms contain a wide variety of learning and behavioral problems and that Erik needed cognitive stimulation and the reinforcement of appropriate social behaviors, listened sympathetically to our desire to find or to create a more imaginative space in which he might continue to re-story his life.

Given this divergence of professional opinion and personal preference, we investigated other inpatient rehabilitation programs along the northeast coast to see if any had additional or different services than those Erik had already received. We visited the St. Lawrence Rehabilitation Center near our home and inquired about inpatient and outpatient options. It was clear that Erik could not return to school in September, but who would oversee and coordinate the therapies he still certainly needed when we left this haven in early October?

The choices facing us about Erik's long-term care, of course, affected all of us. It was as if our entire family system had been shipwrecked, cast into stormy waters, and needed to recover firm ground. For nearly three months, during which time Robert and I gratefully were able to set aside professional responsibilities, we had taken temporary shelter in the acute care hospital and then in the rehabilitation center. These institutions had become island crucibles where we each wrestled with what it means to be human. We had watched our unresponsive child regain motion and some of his senses; we stood by as the wild waves of brutelike agitation beat within him; and we marveled at the enchantment produced by the halting return of language. Each day, on our arising or lying down on the cot beside our son at night, Prospero's words, "We are such stuff as dreams are made on, and our little life is rounded with a sleep," hung in the air around us.

After Labor Day Robert returned to his office in New York for the first time since May. On the 7:17 A.M. train from Wilmington, torn from the son for whom he would have sacrificed his own life, he penned:

Somehow I can't stand the competitive world anymore, where it matters how smart, quick, graceful, suave one is. I need a sheltered world where those qualities are resisted as standards, and handicaps are fully accepted. I don't want to compete. I don't want Erik to have to face competition. Yet the entire academic world is based on competition. I hate tests and performance indicators!

I requested a leave of absence from my college to continue with Erik's rehabilitation at Dupont and then to coordinate the return home in October. Robert's parents arrived to provide stable grandparenting for Sonia as she transferred from the large public junior high school to begin her eighth-grade year in the smaller, private Princeton Day School, where Erik had been a student since eighth grade. Although all the pieces of the plan for Erik's return home were not fully worked out, we had decided to place him in a day rehabilitation program at St. Lawrence Rehabilitation Center. A small group of his school friends had agreed to go to St. Lawrence twice a week in the middle of their day to participate with him in recreational therapy. Extraordinary concern and compassion for Erik—indeed, faith in human potential—on the part of several faculty members and the headmaster at Princeton Day School led to preliminary discussions about whether and how Erik might be able to resume any education-rehabilitation work in that familiar setting. We planned to continue to consult with other rehabilitation professionals and institutions after we were all settled at home again.

During September Erik and I spent five days a week in Wilmington and the weekends at home. He continued intensively with academic and other therapies. He spent longer periods of free time in the gym, dribbling and shooting a basketball, and he was becoming increasingly aware of other patients, sometimes asking what he could or should say to them. Each day his academic therapist and the speech therapist gave him overnight assignments to prepare for the following day. Despite frustration at the painstaking slowness with which he could proceed, he persevered and took satisfaction in completing the challenge. Every challenge required laborious concentration, and Erik met each one with heroic determination.

At the end of the first week in October we mindfully and gratefully said our farewells to each therapist, medical doctor, psychologist, and social worker, and to the other patients who had become a major part of our lives for three months and who had contributed to the fuller second delivery and habilitation of our son. The young teenager who sat beside us now in our car, headed for home, was both the child we had welcomed into our lives sixteen years earlier and a new being who was an unfolding mystery to us. Living within the space between these two human realities presented the deepest challenge of our lives.

The Scattered Self

At home in Princeton Junction
on an October Friday morning,
Sonia anticipated her hope since May:
a return to normal family life.

Robert's parents sent Sonia off to her new school as they had for the past month, and then his mother began leisurely preparations for a festive homecoming meal as his father handily completed several home maintenance chores that had been neglected in our summer's absence. At the Dupont Children's Hospital on our day of departure, each daily act that we had come to perform regularly over the preceding three months I did on this morning with acute mindfulness. We narrated every action together with Erik as we folded his clothes into the suitcase and took down from the walls his name and date signs and the posters that friends had brought him. We walked past particular courtyards or therapy rooms where he had learned to crawl or to speak and expressed thanks to each therapist on his last day as an inpatient.

Going home and coming home. Going home, led by memory, was infused with anticipation that we could make a mythic, eternal return; the other hinted at obscure new realities, threatening us darkly with the truth that we could never go home again. Going home was symbolized by the food-laden table around which human beings universally gather. The aroma of favorite foods welcomed us through the kitchen door and drew us into a cocoon of safety. For three months Sonia, Robert, and I had longed, each in an individual way, for the ordinary routines of summer and for the familial and religious traditions that had previously anchored our lives.

Coming home was something else again. Sitting at the dinner table that first evening, happy that we were all together again, I realized faintly that coming home was not the same as I had imagined going home to be. In the tear-filled eyes of Erik's stoic Danish grandfather as he lifted his head following a grace of gratitude, I read the clues of truth: we were not the same. Though the food spread on the board this evening was familiar, Erik's lost olfactory sense dulled his taste. Gone was the light, often witty repartee that had previously taken place between brother and sister or between father and son; in its place were careful promptings and monotone replies or a glazed stare. Bites that were too large or chewed with his mouth open were overlooked at this homecoming dinner but noted silently with disgust by his sister and with pathos by us, who had been coaching him for weeks about eating decorum. We all tried not to speak too quickly, expect too much of Erik, carry on too many conversations at once, or do anything that we thought would confuse or upset him. The sweetness of the homecoming meal was seasoned with the bitter herb of grief.

At our table that first evening, as we joined together, I realized that I was coming home to a new level of awareness within me. The rehabilitation that had occurred during Erik's three months at Dupont Children's Hospital, which we had celebrated as we closed that chapter, quickly became visibly inadequate for the complex, multifaceted demands of busy professional life in an eastern suburb of the United States.

Were we, by trying to maintain a forward, continuous movement in Erik's life narrative, obscuring from ourselves and the world the real events of disintegration, to which we give little place in our carefully delineated personal stories or in any shared cultural story?[1] Fourteen years later I answer my own question: in the face of overwhelming disintegration, too obvious to ignore, we tried simply to help Erik reorganize the pieces into some coherent pattern that he and others might consider a self.

The first three months following the accident, in which most improvements from traumatic brain injury would supposedly occur, had already passed. Though Erik's gains from total unresponsiveness to the cognitive functionality of a fifth or sixth grader had been remarkable, we lived with the knowledge that his progress could plateau or stop at any time. We also recognized the wide and awkward gap between his chronological age and his social behavior and between his diminished affective expressiveness and his need for human acceptance; we wondered if those gaps might exist as permanent consequences. We had brought our son home to a physical space filled for us with rich textures of memories and aspirations in which he seemed only a skeleton of his former self. He was in some ways like a house deserted while still under construction: the architectural plan had been laid in his genes and our dreams, a foundation lay in the womb of the unconscious, and a framework in consciousness had been taking shape through his childhood development and choices. With the accident and coma, all visible work on his "house" had ceased. Now, back in his family home, some confusing array of biological, psychological, cognitive, and spiritual elements that we still called Erik wandered, in and out among the two-by-fours, the studs and girders, and unfinished floors of his self. It was as if he had been shaken upside down and inside out; sometimes it almost seemed as if "he" had flown out of his house. Could this child's framework ever be filled out with walls and windows and doors, with life-giving water and electrical current flowing to all parts, with rooms for inquiry and reflection, with plentiful touches of beauty and spaces for music and laughter? Could all these ragged and disarranged elements cohere?

The longing to return home and again become a family impelled and sustained us throughout the months from May to October. Many of our activities during the first two or three weeks at home reflected our desire to reintegrate Erik into the intimate family circle and into a wider social community. For example, in preparation for our return, we sent a letter to our near neighbors and friends describing Erik's condition, encouraging them to reintroduce themselves to him when they saw him outside, and informing them that, though he would be sometimes disoriented or impassive, their engagement with him was important for his ongoing rehabilitation. We were trying to normalize and gather the disjointed pieces of a situation that could only be described as shattered. Driven intensely by this hunger for home as we had known it, we planned a two-hour homecoming open house with eight of Erik's close male friends on the first Sunday we were all back together. They all agreed to come to get reacquainted with Erik.

Preparations for the party mirrored those we undertook for leaving Dupont. We asked Erik for his suggestions for the menu, inquired about the feelings he had as he looked forward to being with his friends again, and rehearsed appropriate behaviors. Though Erik appeared pleased that his friends would be coming, he was unable to contribute food suggestions, simply saying that our recommendations were fine, and he seemed unable to project himself forward a few days and to imagine acceptable or awkward behavior. Because he tired easily and was less alert and interactive when tired, we suggested he take a nap before the party, but we gave him the responsibility of arranging items on the refreshment table with our help.

As Erik's friends began to arrive, two people but three sets of feelings greeted them. Erik and I stood together, each expressing genuine pleasure that they had come. I noticed immediately the suppleness of their bodies and the quickness of their smiles and hands, extended for greeting, even in spite of some typical adolescent nervousness. A third voice, audible only in my head, tormented me, insinuating the unfairness of vacations in Europe or along the ocean coast, of tennis games and movies, and of another life—our son's—pulled out of time. These friends, rested from the summer, looked keenly alert for the challenges of a new school year. In contrast, our son had spent his vacation wrestling with death and was lost to himself in disheveled neural nets. In his monotone voice Erik greeted each one and then waited for someone to initiate a movement. Prior to the accident they would have all greeted each other hastily and then bounded enthusiastically to the backyard for catch or upstairs to the computer. Now the boys moved stiffly to the family room and sat in a circle as their parents or grandparents might have done if invited for tea. Either Robert or I, along with one of the boys' beloved Princeton Day School teachers, who had come to the party, stayed in the room to help negotiate the conversation. Soon Erik's friends were talking animatedly about their classes, teachers, and funny experiences over the summer as Erik tried desperately to process all the stimuli coming at him. Occasionally he laughed belatedly or made a bizarre comment which, because it seemed only remotely connected to the present topic, Robert or I tried to tie into the conversation by asking Erik questions or supplying linkages for others. Only when the captain of the football team, who had broken his leg in Friday night's game, arrived with the game ball for Erik did the party relax. On crutches and in a cast, Scott pressed them all to move out to the backyard to throw the football.

Sonia and I watched from inside, she delighted that her brother was back with his friends playing ball and I hoping that a tossed football would not hit Erik in the head or that his slowed reflexes wouldn't land him under someone. The gap between who Erik had been and who he was now widened visibly, but I took little note at the time of the gap between Sonia's joy and my anxiety. When the boys gathered later around the food table, they expressed their admiration for Erik's athletic prowess—a word that seemed at once condescending and supportive—attempting, I am sure, to encourage him in the face of the large obstacles looming before him. Perhaps they genuinely recognized how far he had already come.

Erik could not describe *his* feelings and was incapable at that time of reflecting on the significance of this visit with his friends. Some of his uncoordinated movements, his occasional, random outbursts of laughter, the incongruities between his behaviors and those of his peers, his emotional detachment in this social encounter, and his location on the fringe of this group of friends evoked incredulous, though polite, bafflement from these young men. Erik looked physically like our son, but he didn't act like the boy they, or we, had known. Mentally and socially it was as if his feet were where his hands should have been; from his mouth came comments that were sometimes crude, uncouth, or meaningless.

Initially, the pain of seeing Erik's shattered self prevented me from recognizing how like the classic trickster Erik appeared in his difference from others. Many years later a friend who knows of my interest in tricksters showed me a collection of narrative poems from the Swampy Cree Indians. Opening the book, I read

> I try to make wishes right
> but sometimes it doesn't work.
> Once, I wished a tree upside down
> and its branches
> were where the roots should have been!
> The squirrels had to ask the moles
> "How do we get down there
> to get home?"
> One time it happened that way.
> Then there was the time, I remember now,
> I wished a man upside down
> and his feet were where his hands
> should have been!
> In the morning his shoes
> had to ask the birds

"How do we fly up there
to get home?"
One time it happened that way.[2]

How profoundly this tale metaphorically expressed my view of Erik's present condition and challenges. Tricksters are tale spinners who traditionally preside over change; they live on boundaries or thresholds between one place or condition and another; psychologically they mediate between what the ego wants to hide in social conventionality and the transparency of the self. In their strange antics and befuddling nonsense speech tricksters show us the interpersonal and interactive dimensions of selfhood. In their uncomeliness they remind us that human development never rests in static states but unfolds through dynamic processes.[3] There was no doubt in our minds that Erik was in the process of "going between" one form of existence and another and that he was again passing through developmental stages. The gap between conventional behavior and Erik's sometimes impulsive actions or disconnected thoughts occasionally led to surprising outcomes, but they were consequences of brain injury and not, as they are for traditional trickster figures, expressions of playful cunning or creative experimentation. Nevertheless, comparing the trickster's attributes to Erik's postinjury condition gradually allowed me to respect Erik's bizarreness, to detect the pieces to be refashioned in his own reconstruction, and to engage him in his lostness. The scattered self of our son was introducing us, as the trickster in many cultures does, to the changeableness, the contradictions, and the impermanence of life that we humans seek to control or suppress. If I had focused only on those actions or traits that made Erik different from others and seemed often like an inversion of the ideal personality and "normal" behavior, I would have misrepresented the trickster and left Erik locked outside on the margins of life.

During the first ten days at home and as Erik began his outpatient rehabilitation program at St. Lawrence, we simultaneously tried to set-

tle into a reliable home routine that would order Erik's days and continued to investigate other, long-term, rehabilitation options. Our initial impressions of the St. Lawrence program, plus the information
gathered from four other visits with neuropsychologists and educators,
gradually clarified not only the direction we would take to address Erik's
substantial needs but also our attitudes toward selfhood in general and
his personal story, which we sought to sustain. All our schedules and
needs were subsumed under Erik's rehabilitation. Fortunately, Sonia
seemed to have made a happy transition to eighth grade at Princeton
Day School and was doing well in her classes; I was on leave from Stockton, and Robert was able to work at home several days each week. On
the surface at least, Sonia seemed to take courage to develop her own independence in what seemed like normalcy. Each of our lives became sub-
texts, or perhaps subplots, in the service of the main one.

The St. Lawrence Rehabilitation Center had begun to accept traumatic brain injury patients shortly before Erik began his day program
there. Primarily a facility for stroke patients, who generally were elderly adults, St. Lawrence seemed to Erik, who had just left a children's
hospital, a depressing place. Some staff members, who were adapting
to treatment protocols in the brain injury program, seemed particularly
intent on making Erik confront his significant deficits as a prerequi-
site for developing new strategies. Without a then adequately functioning frontal cortex with which he could initiate and direct his own
actions and reflect on who he had been and was now, he simply resisted their suggestions that he was denying his reality; hence he lived
many of his early days at St. Lawrence on the edge of anger. As his parents, whose persistent hopes for his continuing progress could also be
construed as denial, we did not want to dampen his motivation, so we
found ourselves caught between therapies that seemed predicated on
pessimism and aspirations that we at least dimly recognized might be
unrealistic. Though our deepest hopes remained unarticulated, we still
believed in the restoration of Erik as a unified and only slightly altered

self, provided that he didn't plateau or have other setbacks. An excerpt from Sonia's diary reflects a similar and appropriately adolescent confidence.

Diary, . . . I'm sorry I haven't written to you in so long but I've been over-whelmed. So much has happened. It seems like a lifetime since I did write. . . . Erik is now back to practically normal. . . . But my life is back to normal. God—it took so long for that to happen, but when I write it, it seems like only a little while ago.

With such scarcely conscious beliefs governing our lives, we sought the advice of three neuropsychologists who had been recommended to us; two were affiliated with institutional programs north of us, and one was in private practice near Philadelphia. All three were impressed by the progress Erik had made, and all felt they could offer additional assistance. During my visit to the first facility, the uniqueness of Erik's circumstances registered more acutely on me. The day patients in that program were on average five to twenty years older than Erik. Many were attempting to return to vocational employment, not to school. Many had been injured in motorcycle accidents; some blamed their injuries on alcohol. Compared to Erik, these individuals had been toughened by life experiences quite different from his. The thought of putting Erik, who seemed still so much an impressionable child, into such an environment deeply troubled us.

The second neuropsychologist outlined our two options very clearly: we could place Erik in an institutional setting, or we could create an individualized program. After having been told by some of the Dupont rehabilitation professionals that Erik should be placed in a learning disabilities or special education classroom to complete his high school education, we welcomed the strong recommendation of this psychologist that he not be so placed, at least yet.

After these first two visits we were attracted to an individualized approach, though we were uncertain about who would develop and coordinate such a plan. We and Erik then met Dr. Kurt Ebert, the neuropsychologist in private practice. Prior to our visit he had asked to see the results of psychological and I.Q. tests that had been conducted on Erik after the accident and school essays or reports that Erik had written prior to his injury. After he gathered information about Erik from all of us and explained his professional background and approach, Dr. Ebert met with Erik alone. After his assessment he told us that Erik was performing analytical tasks at a fourth-grade level. We were distressed to hear him report such a discouraging evaluation in Erik's presence. Dr. Ebert proceeded to tell Erik that his friends would want to see the old Erik, but the old Erik is not here anymore. Then he recommended that he work with Erik twice a week on cognitive and psychosocial aspects of rehabilitation. Dr. Ebert became exceedingly important to Erik as together they worked to address the psychological reactions to Erik's injury and to build on his former mental abilities through repatterning exercises that used a variety of neurological and psychological approaches, including neurolinguistic programming techniques. Whatever else we might choose to have Erik do—an institutional day program or tutoring—would simply supplement what Dr. Ebert thought was critical to Erik's cognitive functioning.

Between these investigatory visits, two of Erik's teachers and the headmaster of his school visited on separate occasions. Each of the teachers in his or her own way reached toward the Erik they had known in class. Janet Stoltzfus, who had seen Erik both at Cooper Hospital and several times throughout his months at Dupont, recalled past classroom experiences, talked about his friends and their current activities, referred to novels they had studied, and teased him about his fondness for short journal entries. Whenever Erik gave an indication verbally or facially that he recognized what she was describing, both appeared pleased. When Stephen Lawrence, who had not seen Erik since the accident, came to visit he asked Erik if he could remember Hamlet's "to be or not to be" soliloquy that the students had memorized in his class. Mr. Lawrence began to recite it and waited. Because we had observed that most of the people or events that Erik seemed to recall spontaneously came from at least two or three years prior to the accident, we were amazed when, after Mr. Lawrence began again and waited, Erik continued with a few of the right words and with some imported from another part of Hamlet's speech as well as unrelated words. Both these educators expressed concern for the person trapped inside a tangled brain and were fascinated by the mysteries of the brain's connection to selfhood. Their interest and offers to help in his reeducation met us in our place of deepest need.

A consummate educator of whole children and their parents, Sanford Bing, the Princeton Day School headmaster, arrived for a visit one Sunday morning as we continued to sort out the best long-term plan for Erik's rehabilitation. He listened in the spaces between and beyond our words, he talked with Erik respectfully, and he validated Sonia by telling all of us how glad they were to have her at Princeton Day School. With acute attention to our need and affirmation of our hope, he not only encouraged us to trust our instincts, which were leading us toward an individualized approach to Erik's ongoing rehabilitation, but also offered to assist us in whatever ways he could. He was quick to point out the obvious—Princeton Day School was a private, college preparatory school; it did not have a program or resources for special education— but he wondered if a special education setting was what Erik needed. Though he departed from our house with the simple agreement— possibly no more than politeness—that he and we would stay in contact, he seemed somehow like a messenger of promise.

Interspersed with these visits that, especially in retrospect, exposed our hope that Erik might somehow return to who he was, came phone calls and visits from a rehabilitation nurse hired by the insurance company. She was in the awkward position of trying to support us in our decisions about Erik's needs while also protecting the interests of her employer, the insurance company. She counseled us against denying Erik's deficits and lobbied for drawing on public resources like the special education classroom as a placement for Erik. After such conversations, which agitated more than supported, I wondered how Erik's struggle to reclaim his life was being affected by all who were narrating it from their points of view or interests. My husband was flatly irate and determined that we advocate for Erik's interests at every stage.

By the end of our first month back together as a family we had settled into a fairly regular routine that included a day rehabilitation program at St. Lawrence supplemented by twice weekly trips to Philadelphia to see Dr. Ebert. These arrangements required careful negotiation with the insurance company and interpretation for the staff at St. Lawrence because both, for differing reasons, feared duplication of services. The insurance company, in a no-fault state, surely did not want to pay for more services than were basically necessary, and some of the psychologists at St. Lawrence worried about adding stress to Erik's life by introducing too many therapies at once.

Each day at St. Lawrence included traditional occupational and physical therapies plus individual academic sessions to relearn math and reading comprehension. Once a week over the noon hour two of Erik's friends, driven by one of the parents to St. Lawrence, participated in some form of recreational therapy, a session designed as much for its socialization benefits as for physical ones. This schedule seemed manageable and predictable to Robert, Sonia, and me, but Erik still often appeared lost. Though he was living in his family house and sleeping in his own room, he benefited from our regular and repeated recounting of his daily activities.

Spatial disorientation is a common consequence of brain injuries. For example, we often found Erik roaming from room to room in our house as if looking for something or trying to remember where he wanted to go and for what purpose. On such occasions we tried to jog his own memory with questions and by suggesting associations with a previous activity that we thought might have stimulated his search. At St. Lawrence simply making a left instead of a right turn off an elevator could lead him on a circuitous path to his destination. When Erik went out into the neighborhood or with us into the town or to shopping malls, or even when he returned several months later to his school for tutoring, we often drew maps of the places he would be navigating and always talked through the directions. In all such circumstances we were, in a sense, trying to think both for ourselves and for Erik. We needed to identify the clearest routes to his desired destination and then anticipate how his failure to notice important visual cues in the environment could confuse him. Often we felt like novice mind readers or clueless detectives trying to follow an insubstantial trail of evidence.

Erik's lostness in space did not show up merely as disorientation in physical locations. He was also lost psychologically and confused mentally. Erik's disorientation in space simply mirrored his mental disorientation, rendering social interactions and self-knowledge exceedingly difficult. In conversations this apparent lostness to himself and from others became most visible. Sometimes in the midst of discussion on a topic Erik would insert a thought or anecdote that seemed random—totally irrelevant or inappropriate to the present exchange. Or he might begin a thought and lose the gist of the idea in the middle. One occasion occurred shortly after he had returned home, when one of his male friends from school came to visit. As Erik's friend talked to him about what was going on at school and what he had done in the summer, the friend's mother and I visited on the other side of the room. In the midst of their heavily one-sided conversation, Erik gently put his feelings of friendship into words, baffling his friend. Teenage boys do not generally voice their feelings directly in kind words.

On another occasion the parents of the driver of the car in which Erik had been injured came one October evening to return Erik's book bag, which had been recovered from the vehicle. Erik came down from upstairs to greet them. Instead of a socially conventional greeting, Erik's first words were "I forgive you." From where did these words come? No one had apologized or perhaps even considered forgiveness necessary, but Erik extended it from somewhere out of his own lostness. Erik's higher cognitive functions were still in disarray, so one could hardly claim that the urge to forgive arose from moral reasoning. This forgiveness, offered without guile from a child to adults, was socially astonishing, but to the acutely sensitive it was understood because of its authenticity and transparency. Erik's lack of normal inhibitions, a characteristic of his lostness, moved him toward innocence. His words sprang from some inner reservoir. Robert and I were left in a state of shock: our fragmented son was acting out what we ourselves found difficult to implement even though we knew forgiveness was integral to our religious beliefs. Erik's words, unexpected and forthright, exposed the falseness of the familiar social conventions of hiding resentment behind politeness and of refusing to acknowledge the effects of our actions on others.

Lostness in space and to himself as a space expressed itself in frustration and denial as well. In mental "places" where Erik had previously felt at home—as, for example, in working algebra equations, mastering geometry, or solving calculus and physics problems—he now wandered in confusion as he tried to find his way. Often he erupted in anger against his speech therapist, who doubled as a math tutor, vehemently denying that he was no longer at home in his computational house. Who was he if his former abilities and means of experimenting in and with his world were so compromised? Some outbursts unnerved us all, but they especially affected Sonia, who could be embarrassed by or impatient with his difficulties and wanted him to succeed as much as he did. It became apparent that Erik could not hold multiple strands of conversation in his mind at once and that he had difficulty perceiving contexts fully and instead would attach to only a snippet or single thread of conversation.

Discouragement and depression lurked in the shadows as Erik worked to reorient his life. Occasionally he said, "I'm sorry I've ruined your lives." As we reassured him, saying that what had happened to him was not his fault, we guessed that he may have been feeling the loss of his own life. A few months later when he returned from his day program at St. Lawrence, he reported that the neurologist there had helped him find himself. Once at home he said he didn't like the mixed-up person that he had found. He said that Erik was dead: "Not dead in body, but my mind is dead."

Thanksgiving and Christmas, traditionally times for anticipation and festive feasting, were tinged with poignancy. Six months had elapsed since the accident, and we found that our gratitude for Erik's survival and his dramatic progress was clouded by a sharper awareness of the changes that had occurred and of a future that lay shrouded in uncertainty. Often when we doubted and struggled with these alterations, others glimpsed causes for hope that we could not see. On the day of the holiday assembly at Princeton Day School, Robert, Erik, and I went to see Sonia perform in the chorus. Though not in school himself, Erik was keen to walk into the assembly with his group of friends and to sit with them. They welcomed him graciously, despite his awkwardness and his responses to the confusing overstimulation of so many people, the great commotion, and the excitement that a major holiday generates. As we watched the classes gather the headmaster came to us and exclaimed enthusiastically that he had just heard that Erik was now performing in math and reading at the seventh-grade level, a report we had not yet received from St. Lawrence. From relearning the multiplication tables in September to doing seventh-grade math in December represented significant cognitive progress, and we tried to balance this good news against the pain we felt as we watched Erik, out of the corners of our eyes, try to negotiate his former world.

As our wishes for our son clashed with our increasing awareness of the reality that brain injury imposed upon him, we drew upon any resources, from our intuitions to suggestions from friends and professionals alike, that we thought might have beneficial therapeutic effect in helping to put the roots of his life back into the ground. All who related to Erik were shaping a bridgelike narrative that we hoped might carry his consciousness across the rift between a dimly or only partially remembered past and an altered present. Though I could not explain neurologically why we were doing what we did at the time, I had a gut feeling that all our interactions with Erik and explanations about or descriptions of those interactions flowed like a river to restore some coherence to his life. In the absence of Erik's ability to tell his own story, we learned experientially what Antonio Damasio later described from his neurological research, that "the images in the consciousness narrative flow like shadows along the images of the object for which they are providing an unwitting, unsolicited comment. . . . The story . . . is not told by some clever homunculus. Nor is the story really told by *you* as a self because the core *you* is only born as the story is told, *within the story itself*."[4] While Erik was unconscious we held the images of him and told the stories about him. Now that he had consciousness he continued in our minds as the "object" of our attention and commentary. By interacting with and commenting on him, we hoped to contribute to his capacity to take up his own story.

Arthur Frank's *The Wounded Storyteller: Body, Illness, and Ethics* insightfully elaborates the importance of storytelling for the interpretation of illness experiences. Describing three basic types of story—restitution, chaos, and quest narratives—Frank reveals the body's dependence upon multiple stories or variants of the three types for navigating the terrain of illness. During the three months that Erik had no capacity to tell his own story, we as parents found ourselves weaving elements of these three types of narratives on Erik's behalf. We struggled to reckon with the chaos of unspeakable grief, for traumatic brain injury breaks all familiar coherence to smithereens, and we feared that all order had been destroyed and would not return for our son. To Erik, however, we tried to present stories that linked his former, healthy self with his present, recovering self and that projected a future of restored well-being. Without the ability to tell, Erik's own body-spirit enacted a kind of quest narrative. His determination not merely to survive but also to surmount devastating obstacles continues to bear witness to this quest. Confirming our experience with Erik, Frank makes visible the interactive nature of health and selfhood.[5]

By Christmas 1985 it was clear that we were piecing together, with the able assistance of many professionals and friends, an individualized ongoing rehabilitation program for Erik. As I look back on the period from 1 January 1986 until the summer of 1987 and recall all Erik's experiences and activities during that important year and a half, I now interpret that as a time of house rebuilding. If, as Martin Heidegger suggests in "Letter on Humanism," language is the house of being, Erik was engaged through language, though not language alone, in reconstructing his being.[6] As a self he had to undertake a process similar to his tree house construction project several summers earlier. As he had done then, guided intuitively by some interior desire or directive to build a youthful dream, he now scavenged in his brain for lost but still usable parts. He rummaged through memories with the aid of family and friends for recognitions and connections, he tried out new behaviors or strategies and even ways of clothing himself, and he sought to open blocked or new neural pathways through creative activity. More than simply occupying space, we wanted him, as we assumed he himself wanted, to become an integrated place—a self at home within his story.

Perhaps understandably, given the high priority we as parents placed on the life of the mind and his pre-accident orientation toward academic work, Erik seemed highly motivated to prove to others that he could return to the performance level he had known before his injury. Although everyone admired his determination, a quality often severely impaired in one who sustains severe brain injury, many also considered it laced with denial. As he continued cognitive therapy at St. Lawrence, largely focused on academic relearning, on a gradually diminishing schedule, he began a tutorial chemistry class in our home provided by our public school corporation and a writing tutorial provided by Mr. Lawrence, his Princeton Day School teacher.

Along with these activities we continued to take him weekly to Dr. Ebert, a visit that Erik always anticipated and that often relaxed his robotic uptightness and opened his attention. From the very first visit Dr. Ebert had prescribed finger exercises for Erik to practice repetitively each day, as often as possible; the more often they could be done the better, for they were to help repattern the brain. Each finger on each hand was assigned a number, and Erik tapped out specific sequences over and over, working for both speed and accuracy. He could perform these patterns while riding in the car, sitting at a table or desk, waiting for a therapy session to begin, even as he was going to sleep at night. In his fascinating work *The Hand: How Its Use Shapes the Brain, Language, and Human Culture,* Frank R. Wilson asserts that "the hand is as much at the core of human life as the brain" by examining the evolutionary and cultural significance of the human hand and linking its manipulative and tool-using capacities to "the redesign, or reallocation, of the brain's circuitry."[7] Wilson's investigation of the development of sign language in the deaf and speech in the hearing suggests an essential interconnection between thought and language and the hand. We observed some relationship or communication between the brain and the hand when Erik was first able to speak again and lines from nursery rhymes came forth with relative ease as his hands caught and tossed a soccer ball; we witnessed it later as his wild, uncontrolled scribbles across a page changed to labored letters, paralleling an evolution of his language and thought when he could speak again.

Dr. Ebert's emphasis on the importance of finger activity to the brain supported our observations that essential connections existed between the body and the brain, physical activity and consciousness, and emotion and cognition. We had followed these connections through and beyond coma and believed that helping Erik to become an integrated being—a freely functioning, livable "self house"—required engaging all his senses as much as possible and both the left and right sides of the brain. The left side was already heavily engaged in relearning academic subjects. With the willing support of a master woodworking teacher at Princeton Day School, Erik returned to the shop, where he had crafted a lovely small cherry table as an eighth grader. Mr. Franz patiently taught and guided him again to enjoy the feel of wood, to design a simple canvas sling chair and later a small Shaker-style table, to coordinate his eyes and hands and brain for accurate measuring, to work safely around power tools, and to persevere—if restlessly and despite occasional distractedness—in sanding and sealing, sanding and sealing the wood to a satiny smoothness.

Once a week during this same period—what would have been the second semester of his junior year—Erik met with eighty-seven-year-old Mrs. Bonato, an Italian painter who resided in a retirement community in Princeton. They painted together, she guiding without judgment his eyes and his hands. Though we were pleased simply for Erik to be in her company and to play with color and line as best he could, Mrs. Bonato respected his strong desire to make something representational and pleasing that he could recognize. Often I watched them together, noting Erik's great difficulty in seeing or understanding perspective or in simply reproducing what I thought his eye should see in the picture he was copying. On such occasions Mrs. Bonato sometimes placed her hand over his and together they applied the first brush strokes on the canvas where Erik needed to begin, or she would direct his attention to places left empty, asking for his recommendations for filling them.

When of his own volition Erik sat at the piano or got out his cello, both of which he had largely abandoned after eighth grade, we encouraged his faltering explorations across the keys or with the strings, wondering occasionally to what extent he was imitating Sonia, who was studying piano and viola. For a few months he took piano lessons again, reawakening a rudimentary sense of rhythm and reconnecting body memory through the interplay of his eyes and hands.

In all these activities Erik required careful direction and guidance, which he sometimes accepted compliantly and other times resisted. Gratifying as it was for him to be able to execute algebraic formulas again, proceeding step by step with his tutor Mark Wilhelm, no one knew how he would handle new material or abstract thinking. So far he had primarily been recovering previously stored knowledge or negotiating present-time stimuli. We had been forewarned at Dupont that frontal lobe injuries damage the brain's executive function, essential for initiation, processing and absorbing new data, and reflection. Though Erik did express some emotion, particularly gross outbursts of frustration and impatience, his affect often lacked the finer nuances of empathy or sadness. When not engaged by others he often sat blankly staring into space. Where was he in those times? Was he thinking? How was he thinking?

Did he have any connective affective memories of his early life as a child, or was he at sixteen effectively beginning from nothing? Could he really think without the development or engagement of his emotions?

John Dewey uses the analogy of a perplexed wanderer in *How We Think* to explain some aspects of cognition, suggesting that thinking begins in perplexity, as a "forked-road situation, a situation which is ambiguous, which presents a dilemma, which proposes alternatives."[8] Surely Erik, who was confronted with profound ambiguities, stood at a forked road. Dewey's assertion that "a being who could not think without training could never be trained to think"[9] posed serious questions for us as we wondered if or how our son was thinking or would be able to think. For Dewey, "thinking involves the suggestion of a conclusion for acceptance, and also search or inquiry to test the value of the suggestion before finally accepting it." The natural resources necessary for thinking include "a certain fund or store of experiences and facts from which suggestions proceed; promptness, flexibility, and fertility of suggestions; and orderliness, consecutiveness, appropriateness in what is suggested."[10] We knew that Erik had access to some stored experiences and facts, but his mental promptness and flexibility were seriously compromised, as was his ability to order suggestions clearly or appropriately. Were we wrong to expect that our interactions with him might "train" him to think again? Were we working for the impossible? Probably it was our own curiosity about such questions and our compassion for our son that kept us reaching out toward Erik with touch and questions and stories. One evening our persistence led to an important discovery.

Sitting at the kitchen table at the end of a discouraging day, we listened and watched as Erik moved from indignant outrage about some obstacle he had encountered in a tutorial session toward dejection and resignation. As his demeanor wilted, Robert and I inwardly grieved for him. Something prompted me in that moment to see if he might have the capacity to understand and to care for himself as an object of his own attention. A mental picture of him as a little boy, a third grader, arose suddenly in my mind, so I began intuitively.

"Do you remember yourself as a third grader?"

"Yes, I think so." I suggested he close his eyes to see if he could picture himself then.

"Do you remember where you went to school?"

"Maurice Hawk." He was absolutely right.

"Do you remember how you got there?"

"I walked."

"Which way did you walk? What path did you take?"

"I went down the street and then back on the sidewalk to the school. Sometimes I went through the woods." Every detail so far was correct, and he sat very still and engaged. Robert and I now had closed our eyes as well. So I continued.

"Do you remember who your teacher was in third grade?" Here I expected he might get confused, for he had been transposing friends and teachers from earlier parts of his life into the present, but he responded directly.

"Miss Potts."

"Can you picture yourself as a little boy in Miss Potts's classroom? What did that little boy—you—feel like in Miss Potts's class?"

"I was good in math. Miss Potts gave me extra work." I returned again to the feeling question.

"What did the little boy feel like in the classroom?"

Without hesitation he said, "He was scared." Surprised, and yet not surprised but filled with compassion, I asked, "What made him afraid?"

"That people would make fun of me."

"Did that ever happen?"

"Yes."

"Can you remember when and tell us?"

"When Jonathan got the book about Ferdinand." I was stunned, for I had never heard this story before. Its veracity was beyond dispute, for I remembered that he had taken the story of Ferdinand the Bull, who preferred sitting in a field of daisies to trying to outwit and then gore bullfighters, for a holiday gift exchange.

"Jonathan threw the book on the floor and said he didn't want that stupid book."

"How did little Erik feel?" I asked.

Erik began to cry as he said, "He felt sad and scared." Then he began to sob uncontrollably as I held him, and Robert and I cried quietly with him. When his sobbing subsided, I asked, "Can you imagine taking that little boy in your arms and comforting him? What would you say to him?"

"I would tell him that I love him."

"Can you feel that little boy still living inside you now?"

He waited.

Attempting to move us all back into the present, I asked, "How might that little boy and you now be alike?"

"We both are sad and scared."

"Do you think when you feel sad now maybe you can give yourself the love you said that little boy needed?" He smiled and nodded. I felt then, and now, as if we had witnessed a birthing of compassion.

Though we did not know what the impact of this exchange might be over time, I worried that perhaps the recall of sad memories would compound Erik's discouragement; however, the release of emotion seemed, in the short run, to have dissipated the despair that had troubled the supper hour. A few days later Erik's educational therapist at St. Lawrence called on another matter, and then in passing she observed that Erik had seemed more alert and engaged in their work together the past few days. I reported our recent memory experience and speculated again, as we had while he was still in the stupor of the lightening coma, that emotional agitation seemed to increase consciousness, that consciousness and cognition depend on feeling. It seemed that by tapping images and feelings of himself as an eight-year-old child Erik was becoming more aware of his own subjectivity. This may have been an extension—an internal experience—of our narration to Erik through stories and through bodily touch when he was still in coma. During those moments when he was thinking about his eight-year-old self he was no longer merely an object receiving our feelings and actions; he appeared to *feel* his own consciousness. Many years later Damasio confirmed scientifically what we had experienced anecdotally around our kitchen table: "the strengthening of rationality probably requires that greater consideration be given to the vulnerability of the world within."[11]

As Erik worked to reassemble pieces of his mental house by relearning basic cognitive skills, he continued to be someone new to us, someone we needed to get to know. Often we directly explored his limits with him. For example, as we moved into the fifth month after the accident, Robert and I were acutely aware that Erik's voice remained relatively monotone and wooden. Just as his consciousness and cognition seemed enhanced by feeling emotions and by expressing them, so they might improve by developing the ability to vocalize a variety of pitches and inflections that often reflect emotion. We noticed that though in conversation Erik's voice was a monotone, when we asked him to sing he would at points raise or lower his pitch a bit even though it was off-key. Seizing on that small variation in pitch, Robert persuaded Erik to sing childhood songs with him while standing in front of the bathroom mirror every evening as they prepared for bed. Over and over they would sing (Robert thought the louder the better!), with Robert beating out the rhythm of the song with one arm while raising and lowering his hand to reflect the song's variation in pitch. Erik joined in: "Row, row, row your boat, Gently down the stream; Merrily, merrily, merrily, merrily, Life is but a dream." They started every session with "Row your boat" but sang many other songs that Erik knew so well that he could, almost by sheer force of will, raise and lower his voice with the tune. Though we did not see immediate benefits in his conversation, we were convinced that practicing variations in pitch helped Erik's natural inflections to return. In addition, the bond that grew between father and son when they actually could *do something together* seemed reassuring to both Robert and Erik. Moreover, the singing gave us all a vivid reminder every day that the promise of further healing was still alive if we worked to nurture it.

Erik's speaking voice, though gaining slight variation from the singing of old childhood songs in front of the bathroom mirror with Robert each night, still remained relatively expressionless.

Soon after we arrived home from Dupont Erik changed his style of dressing. He replaced polo shirts and jeans with shirts and ties and casual pants. He appeared oblivious to the savvy advice of his fashion-conscious, now teenage sister to return to more typical teenage dress, persisting in his preference for the more formal look. Realizing that indifference to self-care and severe, generalized depression are often consequences of brain injury, we considered Erik's new taste in clothes remarkable. What it meant psychologically we were left to wonder.

He carried this "professionalization" of his appearance into frequent talk about taking the part-time summer job in the computer store that he had secured before the accident. Whenever we went to the mall he stopped at Microcon to talk with the manager who had hired him. While we did not want to dampen his determination to resume his former aspirations and activities, we tried to redirect his attention to the rehabilitation tasks in front of him and suggested that he wait awhile to add a part-time job to his schedule. Because of the manager's compassion for Erik's situation, her ability to see a simple relationship with the store as potentially therapeutic, and her willingness to talk with the psychologist overseeing Erik's program at St. Lawrence about how to maximize the rehabilitative benefits of employment, Erik returned to Microcon for a minimal part-time job a year after he had returned from Dupont.

Responses and initiations of mercy continued to open toward Erik. During the months that two of Erik's Princeton Day School teachers had been working with him one-on-one, Mr. Bing had been in conversation with Dr. Tamarra Moeller, then the head psychologist at St. Lawrence and a parent of a Princeton Day School student. As September of Erik's senior year approached, Dr. Moeller suggested that Erik attempt a half-day program at the school he loved, combined with continuing academic support two or three afternoons a week at St.

Lawrence. A small core of Princeton Day School faculty apparently en-
dorsed the extraordinary view of their visionary headmaster. Reflecting many years later on why a competitive college preparatory school
would extend itself to a child struggling to reconstruct his house of being, Mr. Bing said, "The question was always in front of Erik and you,
and us because we watched you confronting it: can he or can't he come
back and reclaim something of his former abilities? If there is a question, why not give it a shot?"

The opportunity for Erik to return to Princeton Day School under
these special arrangements pleased all of us, especially Erik. Sonia, who
was now also in the upper school, regarded his regular, though abbreviated, schedule at the school with ambivalence. She was devoted to
her brother and wished for his continuing progress, but she was also a
fourteen-year-old, the newly elected president of her class, and sensitive to her peers' opinions and judgments. It apparently became commonplace for her friends who did not know Erik's circumstances to say to her,
"Is that your brother? Gee, you and he are *so* different." And then she
would try nonchalantly to explain without really revealing all that she,
with him, was going through. Because she recognized his tremendous
needs and our intensive involvement in assisting him, she rarely mentioned her feelings. When we all looked back on that year we realized
how little support she received from us for her own development or for
carrying out her leadership responsibilities.

Everyone recognized that Erik's return to Princeton Day School was
a bold, if not foolhardy, experiment that would use education, both the
academic subject matter and its social context, in the service of rehabilitation. Erik wanted to be treated as a normal student, but he obviously
needed modified expectations, some alterations in requirements, and
monitoring as well as support. It was cognitively impossible for him to
carry more than two academic subjects: the required U.S. history and
an English class. To these he added a fine arts class in sculpture.

The academic challenges were enormous, for now he and we faced
the test of how well he could process new information, not merely re-

trieve previously stored knowledge. Early quiz results in U.S. history were disastrous. Reading assignments took him three or four times as long as the time needed by an average student, and then he often could not recall what he had read immediately afterwards, let alone a week later for a test. Essay assignments left him lost before a blank page, for he did not know where or how to gather scattered thoughts or feelings and launch into a topic. The fatigue factor from laborious mental processing compounded his frustration. When we thought of his return to school purely in academic terms we felt discouraged and nearly defeated. But when we reframed the experiment as rehabilitation, we began to transfer some of the approaches we had used with Erik as he was first coming out of coma to support this new phase of his reeducation. We engaged him in a kind of dialogical approach to all his schoolwork, because it seemed intuitively to us as if Erik needed to find himself, or awaken to himself, in order to process and assimilate information or ideas. Asking him questions that encouraged him to place discrete pieces of any assignment into a larger picture seemed to construct a feeling relationship between himself and the texts or objects he was studying. Until such a relationship was established, no matter how flimsy or conceptually inadequate, he seemed locked away from that which he was attempting to know.

To read a text—a piece of fiction, for example—one must know that he is reading a text. Surely Erik was conscious that he was reading a book; he knew that he had an assignment. What seemed lacking was his awareness of himself reading—and all the feelings, memories, sensations associated with that act. Though the presence of such self-awareness seems obvious to those whose sense of self has not been disrupted, we found that if we read a paragraph or small section at a time with Erik, as he read either aloud or silently, and then asked about the content of what he had read, some critical connection between himself and what he was taking in from the page seemed to be forged or strengthened. We could move gradually from very concrete questions to questions that involved comparisons or contrasts, that invited him to make inferences, or that asked him to imagine himself into the feelings of the character or author. Only as "he" began to awaken into and with the text—to interact with it—could information from it extend his consciousness and make him a reader.

The process of writing essays was even more time-consuming, for it involved first understanding the books on which he was to draw and then considering what he thought about the subject, characters, or themes. As with reading, we worked to construct a narrative about the essay topic and the resources he was to use through questions and answers. Every paper that he turned in was the product of prolonged and often tedious questioning and at least seven or eight drafts. At the time, and increasingly upon reflection, I wondered who was "telling the story" Erik wrote. Whose "story" did his essays tell? For example, underneath a discussion of "Benito Cereno," which had taken him half a day to read, lay a hidden story about re-collecting the pieces of a scattered self, about reconstructing a residence for a lost self.

When one of his teachers suggested he take a fine arts course Erik initially balked at the idea because of his remembered attraction to mathematics. What he learned in his sculpture class, however, contributed tactilely to his cognition. By engaging particularly his sense of touch through his hands, Erik increased his perception of objects in space and of himself in relation to objects. When working on a clay sculpture of an owl from which he would later make a mold, he was unable to see that one side of his owl was larger than the other. Patiently his teacher kept asking him if he could see a difference between the sides of his owl, and consistently he reported that he could not. Eventually she asked him to close his eyes and to explore the owl's shape with his hands, and he perceived quickly that one side was bigger or higher than the other and proceeded to adjust its proportions accordingly.

Whereas we had direct engagement with the academic parts of Erik's daily life, most of his social challenges in returning to Princeton Day School occurred out of our sight. Though his small circle of close friends continued throughout high school to include him for movies or concerts or tennis at school, Erik's abbreviated schedule, combined with his social awkwardness, his slowness in keeping up with typical teenage banter, and peer pressure, which encourages young people to shun anyone who is different, left him alone much of the time. We observed this when we picked him up from school, when Sonia occasionally confided that she'd seen him wandering in the halls, and when Erik himself reported that he didn't really hang out with his friends much at school. In effect, Erik had returned to high school in the body of a seventeen-year-old senior but with the emotional developmental level of perhaps a freshman. He was dependent on his parents even as he longed for independence. He desired the attention and affection of girls he had previously dated or secretly admired. Though only a freshman and the younger sibling, Sonia now had mental flexibility and social graces that placed her far ahead of Erik, making her seem the older child and confusing them both.

Despite these social obstacles, which would have discouraged many young people from persisting to make connections with others and the world, Erik continued to seek out peers and adults he admired. Through observation, imitation, and conversation when available, he floated like a small space probe attached by a line to the main capsule. Perhaps because of his steadfast persistence and his slow but continuing cognitive gains, by Christmas of his senior year Erik's psychologists suggested that going to college the following year—if we could find the right place— might not only *not* be out of the question but rather be important for his ongoing rehabilitation. We were incredulous, fearing that the competitive demands of college were unreasonable, at least in the immediate future. Dr. Moeller understood our hesitations, but she counseled, "If you suppress Erik's competitiveness, he will be a depressed child." Erik was overjoyed, and we began to investigate small liberal arts colleges that might give attention to students with special needs. Based on a visit he had made two months before his accident, Erik was convinced that he wanted to attend Earlham College, a four-year school affiliated with the Religious Society of Friends, if he could. We helped him prepare applications during January, and by April he had received acceptance to Earlham and two other liberal arts colleges.

As the senior prom and graduation approached, Erik felt satisfaction and a degree of commonality with his peers, even though he was residing on the fringes of his class and in a liminal space between the self he thought he had been and the one he was struggling to find or create. He attended the prom, though we drove him to and from it, and was included by the faithful eight in some end-of-the-year parties. Not only would he graduate with his class, but, like them, he was headed to college. Our entire extended families and local friends came to mark Erik's graduation. As Erik's parents we watched the graduation exercises with special gratitude for his small circle of friends, who had persevered in maintaining their friendship, and for the faith and commitment of a small group of educators who, by their responses to one in need, made visible the definition of education: to lead forth or to draw out something that is hidden or latent. Both the underlying assumptions on which this extraordinary educational experiment had rested, as well as the forms of discourse employed in carrying it out, departed significantly from most traditional educational purposes and classroom objectives. Responding to Erik's injured brain and being, educators became more like midwives or healers than imparters of information and knowledge. They attempted to restore or to call forth that which had been scattered or impaired rather than to fill up an empty vessel or imprint a blank slate. They temporarily laid aside or adjusted rigorous, competitive academic standards in preference for encouraging a child, faced with a different set of rigors, to become fully human again. Erik's response seems to bear out what recent neuroscientific research with mice suggests: that damage to the hippocampus area of the brain—the area responsible for memory formation and for knowing where one is in space—can be improved by the environment.[12] I suspect few of these educators knew, as we ourselves barely discerned at that time, that their actions had assisted us in realizing that coming home had little to do with geography or houses but everything to do with forging new connections within an individual body-brain and nurturing strong human relationships adequate for a life-long journey. Though Erik still had miles to go on an uncharted road, these professionals had helped him gather up the pieces of his former self, scattered at the margins of disorder by the accident, and had led him on the essential first steps away from chaos, isolation, and despair.

Improvisational Selves

Erik's plans	to enter college
in September 1987	coincided with
our family's relocation	from New Jersey
to Indiana	in late July.
The move required	more internal dislocations
and separations	along with promise
for more stable,	integrated family life.

Three concerns loomed large in our minds, motivating our decision to move. First, Robert and I assumed Erik's full participation in life would be easier in a less fast-paced commuting environment. Second, the uncertain long-term medical and economic needs associated with traumatic brain injury made a full-time academic position desirable for Robert. Third, Robert and I had read about the high rate of marital failure in families that undergo profound shock and prolonged stress. We sought to give ourselves time to reintegrate our lives as a couple and a family of four. All of us were adapting our lives to the ever-changing needs of

Erik's rehabilitation. The move to Indiana meant giving up a tenure-track academic position for me. For Sonia, who had already endured consequences of her brother's traumatic brain injury, our relocation separated her from friends and school, multiplying her losses.

Deciding to adjust our professional lives, how to sell our house and locate another in a distant, unfamiliar city, and when to move further complicated the routines we had developed for coping with the consequences of traumatic brain injury. More important was our concern about professional support for Erik's rehabilitation. How could we replace the services on which we had come to rely? Though shocking to acknowledge, in retrospect I think the person whose feelings and voice we may have overlooked as we negotiated these transitions was Erik's. This oversight occurred perhaps because Erik's needs had become like our own second nature; indeed, we predicated the move itself on a crude calculation of his and our family's prolonged needs. As I write now I wonder what Erik felt as he sorted through elementary school mementos with us, as we dismantled his room and the entire house for packing, and as we closed the doors of our New Jersey home for the last time. Reflecting in 2000 on that change in 1987, Erik said,

Really, I don't think I was as sad about moving as I would have been if I'd maintained really close friendships in New Jersey after my accident. All my friends were going off in all directions to college anyway. And so was I.

As Erik prepared to leave home, we became still more conscious of the ways we had, since the accident, been re-storying his shattered life, mediating between him and the physical world of time and space, and interpreting his confusions or strange behaviors to him or to others on his behalf. Watching a video of our family recorded during his grandparents' fiftieth wedding anniversary celebration in July 1986, we detected the improvisational character of our interactions with Erik as he shadowed us in and out among guests, seeking support and engagement with others through imitation. Sometimes we were leading him; at other times we followed him, trying to figure out and interpret an action or a circuitous line of thought. Brain injury required all of us to arrange the

materials at hand, to watch for clues to feelings or thought in body behaviors, and to construct decisions and stories without a clear design or
plan. Together we engaged in reciprocal improvisations that reminded
me of a ritually choreographed Amish barn raising.

I still regarded Erik's life as a continuous, though radically interrupted, narrative, but I began to realize that this self was not neatly or
easily reproduced and might not fit into an old plot or even, for a time,
a linear, progressive line. What was only beginning to break through to
me was that *my* preconceived notions about his narrative would have to
crack open to find beauty or meaning in change. While Erik still viewed
his life as filled with potential, I knew dimly that I would at least need
to adjust my thinking in relation to his story, simultaneously accepting
its fracture and appreciating the threads that held it together. By 2000,
when Erik and I looked back together on those early post-accident years,
he expressed himself with refined capacities for reflection and insight.

*In 1987 I was just living life. I realized that, yes, things were more difficult
or may take more time, but I accepted that and believed that my life still had
potential. I viewed my life as an opportunity to help others in proactive and
constructive ways.*

I wondered aloud to him: When did that insight occur? Can you trace
it to anything in particular? Without hesitation he responded.

*Yes. It happened the night I forgave the driver and his family. Now, in
2000, I think that is something you and Dad still have trouble doing. I really think that forgiveness plays a central role in most recovery processes.
Every rehabilitative effort that I went through simply enhanced my functioning, but it was the forgiveness that enabled me to become more fully psychologically integrated.*

As I heard his words and then inserted them into this chapter, questions and mysteries abounded. I did not doubt for a moment the veracity of what he told me or the subtle, though profound, impact of forgiveness. But I am also certain that his awareness of the significance of
his guileless "I forgive you" must have sprung from his cells or the mysteries of his spirit, not from moral reflection.

As Erik's consciousness continued to extend beyond simple or core consciousness, his drive for independence grew in age-appropriate strength. His determination and his high motivation to succeed, which meant proving himself academically, fueled his enthusiasm for college. The fluctuating reliability of his judgments and his impulsiveness, which we had helped him monitor while we lived together, concerned us for his life away from home. In addition, we knew that the prejudice and discrimination he had experienced in the familiar environment of his high school from those who did not understand or were frightened by brain injury would no doubt follow him to the college campus. With the help of Dr. Moeller, Dr. Ebert, and his high school teachers, we weighed the opportunities and challenges that Erik would encounter as he began college, and we concluded that college would contribute both to the normalizing for which Erik, and all head-injured individuals, desperately yearned and to his continuing rehabilitation. It would be a remarkable step in independence. It was a powerful, healthy aspiration in Erik, and one that we shared for him.

Despite Erik's significant cognitive gains between the fall of 1985 and high school graduation in 1987, we knew that continuing cognitive needs remained, for these had become apparent as he labored to master new material in his three high school courses and to initiate and sustain action. The injuries to the frontal lobes had impaired the critical executive skills essential for information processing. For example, the executive skills of attention are used to monitor incoming information, to distinguish the important from the unimportant, to privilege the important and separate it from background noise, to move from item to item or shift back and forth between the important and the less important, and to maintain focus on one item or event or to share the focus among items. Though Erik's attention span had improved dramatically in the past year, he still struggled to hold a focus when multiple stimuli or background noise distracted him. The skills of information processing require perceptual skills that, according to Odie L. Bracy, "are the basic tools for gestalt information. These are the executive skills that attach meaning to the work product of the attentional skills, while at the same time provide motivation and direction back to the attentional skills by influencing the level of importance placed on incoming information."[1] In order to formulate thoughts and implement actions the "executive director" of the brain must be able to engage in the following activities so taken for granted by the uninjured: recognizing, separating, combining, sorting, ranking, sequencing, categorizing, grouping, and synthesizing.

The development of thought and conceptualization as well as the implementation of actions and solutions depend on the chemical and motor-muscular systems of the human body. Both these systems can affect and be affected by the activity of the executive functions. Memory is also essential to thought and action and is dependent on executive skills, for it not only retrieves stored information and incorporates it into current events or thoughts but also is necessary for filing or storing new thoughts and experiences.[2] Conceptualization and action are also affected by emotion. We knew from experimentation and from Erik's neuropsychological work with Dr. Ebert how important the interface between emotion and cognition is. An absence of emotion flattens awareness and cognition. Excessive amounts of emotions like anxiety or anger can overwhelm thinking and choosing. Indeed, thought and action arise from complex interacting systems of the whole human organism.

At the end of June 1987, before we left the Philadelphia area, Erik received another battery of tests as part of a comprehensive psychological evaluation at the Children's Hospital of Philadelphia. The narrative description of Erik in the clinical psychologist's assessment presented a clear picture of what he, and we his family on his behalf, faced at this crossroads.

> From the standpoint of evaluation, I would expect that his coming college year may be extremely difficult. His basic reading, writing, and mathematical skills seem relatively modest for a person entering an excellent Liberal Arts College; he has continuing difficulties with the kinds of rapid, complex intellectual processing basic to most curriculum content. He has experienced difficulty with reading and

memory this past year in a familiar setting and with curtailed course
load, was unable to manage the advanced mathematics course he
initially selected. He plans, he says, to register for only two major
courses initially and this plan is reasonable provided the courses are
carefully selected to challenge but not overwhelm him. Even with the
curtailed course load, I think he will probably need to have available
ongoing tutorial/counseling assistance in areas of preparation, review,
organization and emotional support and guidance. . . . I think it will
be important for him to have the use of a personal computer/word
processor to facilitate preparation of written assignments and provide
general organizational assistance.

Finally, it seems very important that arrangements be made to
provide individual psychotherapy, preferably separate and distinct
from whatever college services may be available. This will be a critical year for Erik because it will involve separation from his family
and familiar persons, the need to establish himself in an academically
and socially demanding college community, and will probably revive
in different ways issues related to his injury of feelings of loss and
difference, self-esteem, etc. I think this is his major continuing need
and that other questions about long-term needs will probably be
dependent on the quality of his adaptation and adjustment for the
coming year.[3]

With this psychological evaluation buttressing our own experience of
Erik's continuing needs, we prepared a medical history, a description of
traumatic brain injury, and supporting documents for appropriate Earlham College faculty and staff, including his adviser, personnel in the
Learning Center, health services, and campus ministry office. We had
numerous telephone conversations about the availability of the academic
accommodations Erik would need and were assured that his special
needs could be served. At the recommendation of Dr. Moeller we contacted Dr. Odie Bracy, a clinical neuropsychologist and director of the
NeuroScience Center of Indianapolis, to investigate his cognitive rehabilitation program. Because Indianapolis was only one hour west of Earl-

ham College, we wondered if Erik might receive some of the recommended psychotherapy with Dr. Bracy.

When we met Dr. Bracy, a direct, gentle, insightful human being,
we were surprised at the central role computers played in his cognitive
rehabilitation work. Based on the similarities between the human brain
and the computer described by neuroscientists, Dr. Bracy had developed
a set of programs for computer-assisted cognitive rehabilitation. Both
at Dupont and at St. Lawrence Erik had used some computer exercises
to increase his attention span, strengthen memory, and process visual-
spatial information. Because these exercises targeted particular problem
areas, Dr. Bracy described the approach as specific. In contrast, his programs were arranged so that Erik could progress from fundamental to
more complex cognitive functions. This hierarchical approach seemed
reasonable. We had noted how brain injury had seemed to take Erik back
to the reptilian brain and how the rehabilitation of his cognitive processes
had moved along an evolutionary path. Experientially we had witnessed
the ways the body and the brain interacted interdependently, moving
from the most rudimentary motor functions to simple consciousness, extended consciousness, and more complex cognition.

When Erik left Dupont I read parts of *The Working Brain*, in which
A. R. Luria describes three functional brain areas, each of which contributes to complex mental activity. Acknowledging Luria's contribution to his own computer-assisted cognitive rehabilitation programs, Dr.
Bracy explained that the brain stem and other subcortical areas regulate
excitation and wakefulness. The second brain area, which "consists of
the surface of the brain extending over the top to the side (temporal) areas
and over the posterior (back most) areas," receives, analyzes, and stores
information. The frontal areas govern "the programming of actions, the
regulation of behavior in accordance with the program and the
verification that the actual behavior is in compliance with the program
and the demands of the task."[4] This third functional unit was important for Erik's rehabilitation because one of the zones of the frontal lobe
governs executive activity like initiating plans and regulating complex

behaviors to carry out the plans. When I read Luria as an uninitiated layperson, and then when I listened to Dr. Bracy's description of his computer programs to assist cognitive rehabilitation, I was awed by the brain's intricate circuitry, which makes extended "conversation" possible and apparently supports an elaborate dance across the brain's units, centers, and zones.

Dr. Bracy explained to us that the brain, though infinitely more complex than computers, has both hardware and software characteristics. He asserted that those functions that are more similar to software will be more easily changed: "to a large extent the attentional skills and some aspects of the executive, perceptual, and conceptual skills are acquired, developed, and programmed . . . and should be amenable to change through experience and . . . therefore . . . to the proper efforts of rehabilitation."[5] Given the impairment of Erik's executive functions, we were encouraged that Dr. Bracy would be working with Erik in conjunction with his college courses.

We arranged with Dr. Bracy and Earlham College for Erik to be driven to Indianapolis every Friday afternoon, at which time he would meet with a therapist to learn new computer programs that he then would practice regularly for the following week. Each client begins his therapy with simple visual and auditory attention skills and moves onward only after he has developed or strengthened the particular skill. Because the programs are not designed to entertain clients, many often complain that they are boring and give up. But persisting in the face of boredom is essential for retraining attention, according to Dr. Bracy. When the basic skills of visual and auditory attention have been achieved, clients move on to a hierarchically arranged set of programs that include simple to complex tasks focusing on visual, spatial, and sequential skills and verbal memory work, plus problem-solving exercises that require logic, reasoning, and strategy development skills. Dr. Bracy told Erik that he would receive the greatest benefit from the programs if he would devote at least one to three hours daily to practice. This would require determination and discipline in the midst of a busy college life.

Initially I was concerned about how I would have time to do what Dr. Bracy recommended because I had elected to take a full load of courses. But once I began to use the programs, I experienced success that was motivating.

Getting the educational and rehabilitation programs in place before Erik left home helped us as parents in the short run as much as Erik, for we sometimes, especially in the middle of the night, anxiously questioned the wisdom of releasing our special child to a larger society. For over two years we had been anticipating and interpreting Erik's needs; we had tried to enter imaginatively into his confusions so that we might find "him" there and assist him, if possible, through whatever internal mazes he confronted; often we felt as if we were attempting to think for ourselves and for him. We had brought him home to family, neighborhood, religious and school communities and had concentrated on creating or giving meaning to all our shared activities. In short, we had raised him from infancy a second time. Though we chose to use all available approaches to enhance Erik's rehabilitation, including the computer programs focused on information processing, I wondered who would assist him in applying his strengthened cognitive skills to the making of meaning through feelings and imagination, through shared language, metaphor, and symbol, and through the respect and patience that are experienced in community.

As we said our early September good-byes to Erik on the Earlham College campus and began the four-hour drive home, the grief of separation and the uncertainty that letting go always brings were ameliorated by Erik's great joy, despite some anxiety, about his ability to go to college. Regardless of the obstacles he probably denied and would eventually face, he was, I assumed, experiencing some convergence between his former feeling of himself and his present self.

When I arrived at Earlham I believe I was just living. I wasn't thinking about former and present selves. I viewed Earlham as a safe place, a sort of "rehabilitation playground," though I knew I'd have ups and downs and difficulties and that maybe it wouldn't be perfectly safe. I felt a little lonely or alone after you left, but I wouldn't say it was anything out of the ordinary for new college students.

Driving northward through the flat Indiana countryside after leaving our extraordinarily vulnerable son, I once again protected myself from being swallowed into the great hole I felt in my heart by creeping into a reflective, philosophical mode. I reasoned that the self-reconstruction project in which we had been so intimately involved needed to change for Erik's continuing development. Our level of concern did not diminish—indeed, perhaps it heightened—but the engagement and expression of our concern and our interactions with Erik now formed a new variation on the familiar theme of the re-storying of a son. What was occurring within, to, or for Erik was now relayed to us via daily phone conversations. We strove to detect what Erik was experiencing by listening in the spaces between words, just as we had learned to read between the lines of Erik's actions when we were together.

Shortly after we had arrived in Indiana we had sought out Dr. Paul Macellari, a local neuropsychologist, who became over the years an influential psychotherapist and mentor for Erik. With keen insight into both the neurological dimension and the psychological effects of traumatic brain injury, Dr. Macellari confirmed before Erik left for college that there were four intertwining areas in which he struggled to find, reclaim, or reconstruct himself: the cognitive-intellectual, the psychological-social, the spiritual, and the vocational. To be sure, these are the developmental concerns of most young adults. Typically, though, most meet the challenges in each of these areas with strong body-brain foundations on which they rely as they erect and furnish their personal dwelling places in the world. As had been the case from the outset of our journey with brain injury, each of these areas was tied to the others, and all depended on the fullest possible functioning of Erik's executive skills.

Erik's first year was very difficult academically and socially. For example, his conviction that he wouldn't need tutorial writing assistance softened after his first humanities essay. Our regular phone conversations often concentrated as much on helping him formulate his ideas and ways to support them for his writing assignments as on simply encouraging him or upholding him in times of great stress. His roommate seemed kind but not inclined to befriend Erik in any very personal way, and his casual style and preference for disorder in their shared physical space contrasted sharply with Erik's need for order, organization, and a regular schedule for optimum rest. From Erik's reports it seemed as if he spent most of his time alone studying and practicing his computer exercises. Several times during the first half-year he telephoned in despair, begging us to come and take him home. Discerning at those times whether to respond to his request or to elicit the story behind his feelings and discouraging experiences proved exceedingly difficult. How much challenge could he tolerate? At what point might loneliness or rejection overwhelm him? During these phone calls we listened carefully, asked questions, tried to reflect Erik's responses so that he might see his situation from another angle, and invited him to imagine various options in addition to coming home. Not only did we try to feel into his psychological states and to help him feel himself in them, we also confronted on those occasions our own unresolved grief for him and our uncertainty about how to parent a first-year college student coping with brain injury. Over the telephone lines with Erik, in our deliberations about his latest crisis, even in our sleep and dreaming, we improvised a dance of guiding, responding, mirroring, alternating always between leading and following, often hovering near collapse. In the midst of writing about those sometimes agonizing conversations I wondered how Erik recalled them and regarded them.

I think you did the right thing on those occasions when I said I wanted to come home, for if you hadn't I may not be where I am now. To me this illustrates that as a unit we were just living life. Retrospectively, I think such occurrences may have forced you to view me with normalcy.

Throughout the first two years of college Erik still longed to return to things he had previously loved. He enrolled in a symbolic logic class, despite our reservations, because the mathematical aspects appealed to him, but dropped the course, discouraged and defeated, after a few days. I remember his anguish and profound dejection as he cried into the telephone, "If only I had lost an arm or a leg, then people could see that something has happened to me. Because I look normal, they cannot see what I am struggling with. They just think I am stupid."

The fear of being regarded as stupid commonly afflicts those whose cognitive processing has been slowed by serious brain injuries. In a society that values speed, especially among adolescents and young adults, for whom peer approval is essential, any behavior that sets one apart from the norm threatens one's well-being. Additionally, the readiness to pass quick judgment on others without knowledge of their circumstances reveals a pervasive intolerance of differences. Erik expressed his hunger for acceptance and affiliation in the present by mentally and emotionally calling upon the past. In a class notebook he scrawled:

I need to feel my P.D.S. high school friends. I need to reestablish connection with them. They've been with me through the good times and the bad. That's what I need. Someone who remembers. I think I am cutting my bonds, but I had some very good friends there. I can't and don't want to cut all of them or really any of them out. I'm their inspiration . . . or I was. Don't forget fellas in the East. I'll try and make contact in a letter to their home addresses.

All his academic courses required intensive study—taking notes, reading assignments multiple times, reviewing the note cards that he made for drill, working over many drafts of papers with a writing tutor. When he tried to work quickly, as was his pre-accident custom, or to take tests without asking for extra time he experienced frustration and disappointing results. As he gradually accepted and relaxed into the cognitive constraints within which he needed at that time to work, and as he refined his strategies for organizing material and studying, he discovered that he was more successful. One small success could sustain him and reinforce his discipline for several days, and step by step, day by day, course by course, he became an average student.

When he came home for his first fall break six weeks into the school year we were impressed by small but significant changes in his cognitive abilities. He seemed better able to maintain interest in conversations that were not focused solely on present, concrete details. One evening we got together with close family friends who also had college-age children. The conversation was animated and wide-ranging, the banter spirited. Though I could see the effort Erik had to make to follow conversations in which several people were intensely engaged, and even though he primarily followed the verbal volleys in silence, this evening he hesitantly inserted some thoughts into the discussion, which revealed his increasing ability to stay on the topic with others. During that same visit, and increasingly during the following months, we found that sometimes he evinced a surprising insight into our feelings or about his experiences at school. For example, he began to caution us against being overly protective of him, and when I expressed concern about the effects of his roommate's sloppiness, Erik interpreted their differences with unusual understanding: "Mom, he just has a different style."

Over his four years at Earlham College Erik experienced highs and lows in his academic performance. Nothing came easily to him, with the possible exception of some computer classes that he took. His grit as a student shone forth when he attempted to meet the collegewide foreign language requirement for graduation. Erik did not want to inquire about whether that requirement might be waived for him because of his brain injury. Instead he decided to take a summer-long intensive Spanish course at the University of Notre Dame between his sophomore and junior years. This required three hours of class in the morning, time in the language laboratory in the afternoon, and homework and memorization in the evening. Learning a new language under optimal conditions calls for commitment and diligence; facing language study with Erik's circumstances taxed all his cognitive capacities. The first two weeks were exhausting and the results discouraging, for every new assignment built on mastery of the ones preceding it. On the verge of resigning himself to defeat, Erik decided to speak with his professor and to disclose, instead of hide, the limitations with which he was coping.

Being upfront about brain injury in this situation was okay, but in other situations, like employment or even with some educators, people may not be willing or able to understand the particular needs of someone like me. On this occasion, the risk of telling my truth turned out all right. I needed to have another person's interest and support, other than my parents, for my succeeding.

The professor proved to be not only sensitive to Erik's needs but also very able to suggest strategies and adaptations for his approach to language study. They became allies in learning, he finding ways to memorize vocabulary and understand grammatical forms and she gaining insight into some of the intellectual consequences of brain injury. Erik became remarkably successful in the class and satisfactorily completed his college language requirement.

Her concern and support helped me to dive into memorizing and to spend more time in the language lab. Of course, what my experience suggests is that probably all people do their best work when they feel supported.

Beneath Erik's confession about the risk required to tell his professor about the obstacles he was trying to surmount lies a pervasive concern that springs from society's disregard of anyone whose needs or abilities place them temporarily or permanently outside accepted norms. This professor could have thrown up her hands and claimed that she had not been trained to help Erik; some professionals might have become intimidated and simply ignored his admission and request for help. The more Erik's self-awareness expanded, the more profoundly he wrestled between risking disclosure and choosing the apparent advantages of silence.

The psychological development that occurs and the social relationships that form during college are as important as the intellectual accomplishments of students. The challenges in the psychosocial realm to which Erik frequently referred, often only obliquely through frustration or despair, lay in his own emotionality, his interpersonal relations, and his efforts to understand his own sexuality and to find love that would give his life meaning. Compared to typical college students, Erik had a flat affect, stiff physical movements, and slow speech. Very desirous of making a favorable impression and being included in social activities, he sometimes put others off with his eagerness or anxiousness. He was slower than most to pick up subtle cues of either acceptance or rejection and so might persist in hanging around others who were indifferent toward him. Though physically attractive and unusually kind, Erik doubted himself and his worth, especially in competitive contexts. Because all human beings need affirmation of their existence and support for their endeavors for their psychological maturation, deficiencies in those important areas, or diffidence with which affirmation and support were extended, inevitably influenced Erik's redeveloping sense of self.

A small number of faculty and students who learned to know and respect Erik during his four years became, perhaps unwittingly, partners in Erik's self-reconstruction project. Their willingness to clarify something confusing in an assignment for yet another time or to ask him how things were going and then to listen confirmed Erik's sense of self-worth. The variability of Erik's judgment combined with his age-appropriate wish to be sexually appealing to others made him vulnerable to being used or manipulated, particularly by young people whose own characteristics of judgment and needs for affection and approval were in formative stages. Though Erik confided that he was sometimes confused by his peers' intentions toward him or their interests in him as a friend, he was able to form a few close, mutual friendships at Earlham. One male friend, an intelligent Indian premedical student, became Erik's roommate for two years. His medical interests plus his gentle human sensitivity made him curious about Erik's circumstances and supportive of his efforts to make his way through college. Because the boundaries between Erik's desire for others' friendship and his own needs (for regular rest, for order, for quiet to aid concentration, for feelings of efficacy) blurred easily, occasionally Erik found himself serving the needs of his friend to his own detriment. But when frustration about typing his roommate's papers led to his awareness of the cause of the frustration, and the awareness led him to express his frustration to his roommate, he took another significant cognitive and psychological step in his feeling of himself.

During Erik's junior year he met a female student who became a good friend whom he, and we as well, grew to love. Extraordinarily capable intellectually and perceptive psychologically, this friend offered Erik respect and interest. Two of many qualities that attracted Erik to her were her candor and integrity. She was unpretentious in her brightness; her devotion to her family and compassion for their struggles were impressive and surely appreciated by Erik. Both Erik and this young woman had experienced loss or reverse in their lives, and, I suspect, each saw his or her own desire to surmount difficulties mirrored in the other. All such reflections from the outside are highly speculative, of course, and far less significant than the care and gentle love that was apparent when we saw them together. In this relationship Erik's emotional life became more fully awakened, and it had far-reaching consequences for the ease with which he lived in his body as well as for his mental ability to initiate, plan, and carry out decisions. This relationship, which lasted for six years, was an invaluable preparation for his subsequent, permanent relationship. This young woman's care for Erik taught me to see my son through the eyes of someone unencumbered by regret.

Throughout college, while taking in and processing classroom information, negotiating human relationships and loneliness in the dorm or cafeteria, and experiencing the joys and confusions of his deepening affection for a few friends, Erik continued his weekly cognitive therapy and the daily practice of his computer exercises alone, largely out of sight. In some ways these practice exercises in virtual space became his brain's gymnasium. They paralleled Erik's daily life in physical space, where he had to shift his attention from narrow to wide focus, where he sought his way through mazelike conversations or ambiguous social interactions, where he struggled to solve academic or personal problems one step at a time.

As the computer programs neared completion they focused on higher level problem-solving challenges. I became frustrated both by the difficulties some

of the programs presented and by how much time they were taking. I ration-
alized that I could make better use of my time doing homework, so I resisted
continuing to completion. Despite my parents' encouragement, I refused. But
when you [parents] gave up badgering me, then I decided to complete them.
Now in 2000 I believe this simply reveals that I had to choose to do this on
my own terms.

Though I have no doubt that the rehabilitation exercises carried out
in cyberspace contributed to cognitive gains not only during his work at
the NeuroScience Center but also beyond his graduation from Earlham,
they did not address Erik's interest in and need for an interior connection to some spiritual reality that might help him integrate psychologically the past and the present. Many years after his college graduation I
discovered a saved note he had left for the family when he returned to
Earlham after a vacation at home. Reading it now in the silence of ten
intervening years, I can hear the determination to live life forward with
a haunting search for the past.

> *Dear All,*
>
> *Thank you so much for your confidence and support. I am having diffi-*
> *culty accepting less than perfect in myself and in my work. I am leaving*
> *now and I will call you this evening. I will/may/would like to get some*
> *work done on dialog and exercise 5. I love you all.*
>
> *Erik*
>
> *P.S. As I was leaving I said "Bye house. You've been a good house." I*
> *looked at the photos of Sonia and I as children and felt very sad. I also asked*
> *myself where has that young boy in the picture gone? I seem to have lost*
> *him at age 15 or 16.*

Perhaps because religious values and practice had been central to our
family life throughout his childhood, Erik sought a path toward some
kind of integration through inward silence. Though he was not always
enthusiastic about attending meetings for worship or a house church fellowship when he was a child, from our association with the Society of
Friends he had learned about the importance of silent meditation, of

waiting in the Light of God's presence. Dr. Ebert had also instructed him in some nonreligious, meditative interior visualization practices. Together he and Dr. Ebert had created a mental image that Erik could call upon to calm him or to help him focus when his attention scattered; he also could speak to this interior object and "listen" for a response when he got upset, became confused, or wanted simply to sort out his feelings or thoughts.

From his first weeks at Earlham College Erik regularly attended the Friends Meeting for worship, finding there, largely among the adult members, a welcoming and supportive community as well as nurture for some inward experience of God or the divine within himself. Even simply entering the Clear Creek Meeting House produced a quieting effect, Erik said. When he subsequently informed us that he had asked to become a member of the Religious Society of Friends we were not surprised, though he said, perhaps expecting surprise from us, "People might think it's strange that I would join the group that I was with when I got hurt, but I feel this is what I want to do." His initiation of this request pleased us for at least two reasons: he had made the choice on his own, and the decision suggested an awakening of or a responsiveness to a spiritual reality within him. His college adviser, Anthony Bing, was a member of the Society of Friends and a significant mentor for Erik, so Erik undoubtedly discussed his interest in the Friends with Tony. Erik had to write a letter making his request, prepare a faith statement that would be read by a clearness committee, and then discuss his statement and his intentions with the committee. Whenever we visited Erik at Earlham we attended the Clear Creek meeting with him. On every occasion I was impressed by the stillness, the groundedness, that Erik exhibited in that place and among the silent worshipers. I cannot document its rehabilitative effects empirically, but I do think the experience of expectant waiting in silence contributed profoundly to Erik's spiritual-psychological integration.

Although at nineteen Erik described his interest in the Society of Friends largely as his need for a community, the distance of a dozen years revealed a deeper need.

All I recognized at the time I joined the Friends was that just being in the building had a calming effect on me. Also, when everyone around you is focused on the inner Light, that supported my own sense of a force or a Light, or an inner voice, inside me. Maybe some people would call that the unconscious, but I felt it as an inner voice. Brain injured people need to rebuild their identities. In order to do that, I needed to find a base out of which to reestablish my life. When I waited and worshiped in silence, I felt part of something greater, and I needed that to sustain my identity.

In my retrospective view Erik's ability to reestablish his identity among the Society of Friends suggests that an individual's identity is fundamentally dependent on community, despite the individualistic orientation of many psychotherapeutic and rehabilitation approaches. For Erik, the Friends became another family, one that he selected and by whom he was accepted. Without implying causal connections between his membership in the Society of Friends and subsequent choices, we found Erik more willing to experiment with new activities like singing in a college choral group during his final year and being treasurer of a local chapter of the Fellowship of Reconciliation. His awareness of and interest in others and his capacity for reflection deepened. In phone conversations he began to ask us about current international issues or to tell us when he came across an article or book that he thought might interest us, despite the possibility that he might not recall the details of the article. His association with the Friends also influenced his search for a vocational path as he neared the end of his four years at Earlham.

Robert and I, Erik's adviser, and some of his counselors had advised Erik, unsuccessfully, to take five or even six years to complete his college education. His high motivation, his insistence on proving himself, or his sheer compulsiveness made it feasible for him to graduate in four years, but then he, and we with him, had to face the large question of what he could do professionally with a B.A. degree in psychology. From the completion of high school onward, Erik spoke about wanting to help others who had to face struggles similar to his. We understood and admired his desires but doubted the wisdom of the prolonged and sustained graduate education that was required to work professionally in most health services. Once, when he had expressed his service interests, Dr. Macellari had mentioned a then relatively new and growing field called rehabilitation counseling, which required a master's degree. Quite independently, as he had done in joining the Society of Friends, Erik found a program in rehabilitation counseling at the University of Kentucky. When he went with his girlfriend to visit her home in Kentucky during his senior year, they stopped in Lexington so that he could talk to the director of the program and gather more information. He had also considered library science as a possible profession because of his need and respect for orderly systems and his interest in computers. There too he could help others.

As Erik faced these choices in his last half-year at Earlham College, Robert and I realized that what had begun as a continuing rehabilitation experiment had evolved into Erik's search for meaning and life purpose. He exhibited great uncertainty about his vocational decision, waffling back and forth between the two options. One evening he firmly informed us by phone that he had decided to go to the University of Kentucky program in rehabilitation counseling. "I think if I don't enter this program I will always wonder if I could have, and if I could have and didn't I will feel that my potential for helping others wasn't reached." We had misgivings about his choice, which were based on the intellectual demands of graduate study, living in a large university where he knew no one, the eight-hour distance from home, and his social and emotional vulnerability, but we also wanted to honor his independence and desire to translate his own suffering into service. Erik applied and was admitted to the program.

College graduation again brought the extended family together in celebration of Erik's achievement. Only his family, his professors, and a few friends knew how hard he had worked to come to this moment. As we sat on the campus mall under the silent, stately trees and listened to the choral group with which he was singing for the last time, I realized that there was some mysterious transfer under way. Though I knew that he continued to need our assistance and guidance, I had been prevented by my anxiety for his future to look beyond the present moment. I realized that he had already flown from our hands, which were still cupped to support or to protect. I felt an intimation run throughout my body that he was now leading our improvisation, and I was not sure how we would follow.

Between August 1991 and October 1993 Erik not only rigorously prepared for his vocation but also strove to be fully human against all odds. In those years, as he had throughout the years since his accident, Erik believed that being fully human meant feeling normal; feeling normal depended on being regarded as normal by others and being independent. Underneath or perhaps surrounding these two desires common to every young person's ego, I found from time to time a hint of something else taking shape or unfolding in him. What continues to amaze me about these years in Erik's life is the strength and persistence of his drive to know and to express himself.

Erik's efforts to be independent often brought Robert and me into conflict with him. What seemed comfortable to us did not always seem reasonable to him. As we had when he enrolled in college, we advised him to take a reduced load of graduate courses at Kentucky. He listened respectfully, considered the advice of the director of the program, and then registered for a standard load. He argued, "Many students in the program have full-time employment and still are able to manage the course load; without a job, I could devote full time to study." When he received housing information we thought that a room in a dorm that had a dining hall and was centrally located to his classes and the library would be preferable to a more distant apartment. Reflecting recently, he reminded me again of the clarity of his preferences.

I was excited about living in a graduate apartment but appeased you both by asking for one close to the main campus and along a bus route.

When we helped him move to Lexington we unloaded the car and together set up his apartment; we then joined him in locating grocery stores, walking the route from his apartment to the campus, finding his classroom buildings, contacting the local Friends Meeting, and, most important, talking with the director of the program and the office support staff, whom we hoped would be attentive to him.

Although the academic work remained significantly challenging for him, Erik's Earlham experience made him willing to seek assistance from a writing center in preparing papers. He had learned that he needed frequent repetitions to remember new material, that fatigue weakened his mental alertness, and that organization was essential for keeping track of everything, not simply his schoolwork. One important factor distinguished the rehabilitation counseling program from his undergraduate study: the purpose of this program was to educate people to assist those with disabilities. Some of the students, like Erik, had been led to this field by their own disability or experience of rehabilitation. Thus, Erik found general acceptance in the program at Kentucky.

Throughout his twelve months at the University of Kentucky we maintained almost daily phone contact, and in critical times of stress this contact was more frequent. Often these calls became work sessions as he struggled to develop a paper topic; sometimes they were therapy sessions as he vented frustration or disappointment or as we needed reassurance that he was getting along all right. Generally we were eager to hear a summary of how he was feeling and what he was thinking; always we intended to uphold him and, from a distance, to care as intently as possible. Though Erik usually expressed gratitude for these conversations, he sometimes became impatient with what he perceived as our long-distance directives and characterized as our efforts to control him or not to respect his independence. On such occasions our improvisational interplay hit a glitch, and we stumbled to follow his lead when we felt he was not appropriately attentive to details or consequences. He faltered, resisted, or refused to follow our lead when it appeared that doing so would compromise his independence or his drive for personal efficacy.

Often Erik's yearning for independence was prompted not by a conflict between his and our perceptions of his capability or by willful rebellion but rather by a passionate urge for connection or expression.

One February weekend Robert and I looked forward to visiting Sonia, now a sophomore at Earlham, to see her perform in a theater production. We knew Erik had traveled by bus to Earlham the previous weekend to see his girlfriend. As we stood in the lobby waiting for the doors to open for the Friday performance, up behind us came Erik and his friend. Shocked simply to see him when we weren't expecting to, we were dumbfounded (with a lot of anxiety and some anger tossed in) when he informed us proudly that he had rented a car and driven the four-hour distance from Lexington. I have no doubt that loneliness and his desire to be with his girlfriend again, as well as to see Sonia perform and to visit with us, inspired his decision. Though Erik had a valid driver's license and had driven around our hometown area and with us on longer trips, we would not have advised him to make such a long trip on unfamiliar interstate highways alone. Throughout the entire performance that evening, both Robert and I tried to process our individual responses to what we considered an impulsive act. As we talked with him about his decision after the performance, undoubtedly deflating his feelings of accomplishment, he explained how carefully he had prepared for the trip. In 2000 he recalled this interaction poignantly.

I had read maps, selected the best routes, wrote out directions for myself, compared rental car prices, decided on a larger car for safety, checked and rechecked the weekend weather forecast, and stopped whenever I felt strain.

Our differing perceptions of the same event led to contrasting labels for his actions: impulsive versus careful. Anxieties about how he would get back to Lexington safely, questions about whether one of us should accompany him back and then fly home, and a barely discernible inner guidance to trust him overshadowed the whole weekend. As we parted Sunday, he headed south to Lexington in his handsome rental car and we north to South Bend, we faced once again the dreadful need to surrender our caring control.

Mom, what you have reported is accurate, and what I experienced from this my first solo trip was indeed a sense of accomplishment. You and Dad attempted to deflate it and "put me back" in your image of what you thought

I could do. Despite all such efforts, no one could take away the sense of achieve-
ment I felt in having traveled independently and successfully. I felt often I
was getting mixed messages. On the one hand, my parents would remember
things I could do capably before my injury and wish that I could do those
things—like driving—in my present situation. I believed that this trip to
Earlham would make my whole family happy and pleased. Instead they were
concerned.

Erik's understanding of his parents, despite his disappointment in our
reactions, demonstrated his emotional health and unconditional love—
qualities that confirmed his psychological maturity.

As Erik neared the successful completion of his master's program in
rehabilitation counseling he informed us that he had asked the program
director if he could seek an internship, which was the concluding program requirement, at the Rehabilitation Institute of Chicago. When he
was told that he could, he contacted someone at the Rehabilitation Institute who encouraged him to send a detailed letter of introduction and
application. Why did he want to go to Chicago? Why complicate his life
with another move now that he was familiar with Lexington and could
readily secure a placement there? He responded that he knew the institute to be an excellent rehabilitation center and that his neuropsychologist, Dr. Macellari, had been associated with it at one time. We tried
to weigh the pros and cons with him, including our plans to be in Cambridge, Massachusetts, during the time he would be in the complicated
urban context of Chicago, and reminded him that he didn't need to
prove his worth or ability to us. Our questions and cautions were un-
persuasive, so we listened and responded to several drafts of his application letter.

Some feeling *within* him seemed to be leading him to test his abilities
or perhaps to attract the respect of others. He lived safely in Chicago for
a semester and made a few friends through work, he completed his internship successfully, he received the master's degree in rehabilitation
counseling, and he began an externship under the supervision of Dr. Macellari at South Bend's Memorial Hospital in January 1993, while we

were still in Cambridge. These actions challenged our tendencies toward caution, uncertainty, and fear, all sticky residues of grief. Increasingly the autobiographical narrative that Erik was making through his choices, his academic preparation, and his relationships was moving beyond the one we had known and were still protecting. Over the next several years these two stories—ours and his—would continue at times to run comfortably together and at other times to contradict each other sharply.

Our concerns for Erik's present and long-term welfare were not groundless, as we discovered when he returned to South Bend and his first professional employment. Because the hospital externships were usually held by Ph.D. students in neuropsychology, Erik—with his background in vocational and rehabilitation counseling—did not exactly fit the position. His uncertainties about his own abilities, combined with less defined expectations than academic programs provide, his difficulties with initiation and follow-through, and his tendency to compare himself with others often made him anxious. When he was impressed by the testing skills of a Ph.D. graduate student, for example, Erik concluded that he would need to do doctoral study to become equally competent. Dr. Macellari helped Erik appreciate his contributions and reminded him repeatedly that self-acceptance and a calm inner focus promoted optimal functioning. During the first six months of his externship he lived alone in our family house, which compounded the difficulties of adjusting to the world of employment, though theoretically he liked the independence he had. As previously, our regular phone conversations often concentrated on creative problem-solving around job-related issues, responding to his plans for a small group meeting, or simply listening and exploring his anxieties about his adequacy. In addition to our regular phone contact, simple gestures of friendship like rides to work on snowy days from a church friend or an invitation to lunch by his superiors all contributed to the re-formation of his self-esteem.

As his externship drew to an end, he learned that a regional sheltered workshop for persons with mental or physical disabilities needed a vocational evaluator. His degree in rehabilitation counseling plus his recently acquired rehabilitation counseling certification made him an attractive candidate. We role-played a job interview with him several times, and he was delighted to be chosen for the position. He looked forward to being mentored on the job by the man who had interviewed and hired him. Erik's responsibilities included vocational testing to determine the readiness of a candidate for the workshop, writing reports of his test results, and orally presenting his recommendations to the team of case workers, the workshop job coach, and family members. Unfortunately, as Erik was beginning his employment, the supervisor who had hired him left, leaving Erik without a mentor and the facility he had just joined in a state of transition.

The challenges in this position were sizable, even for a person without the effects of brain injury. During the two and a half years he was employed at the workshop there were numerous staff changes and internal shifts in accountability lines. Paradoxically, though this was a workplace philosophically and practically committed to assisting those with developmental disabilities, some on the staff with whom Erik had to work most closely were not always understanding, or even respectful, of Erik's efforts to compensate for his own difficulties of thinking flexibly or quickly on his feet. From the outset, since the person who hired him had left, no one felt responsible to give Erik guidance in doing his job. Instead, because he had an advanced degree and certification, those without these achievements expected him to know exactly how to do things and waited for him to make mistakes. With his keen sensitivity to vibrations from others, Erik detected this lack of support though he had little understanding of all the personal and institutional factors contributing to it. Erik could sense interpersonal tensions, but he tended to assume that something he did or who he was had produced the reactions he received, even when he was not responsible for others' unconstructive attitudes. The organizational and personnel realities of the workplace combined with Erik's tendency to assume responsibility for others' attitudes made this beginning employment rocky.

The two most demanding parts of Erik's job were preparing written summaries for each client and presenting these reports orally in team meetings. He began writing his reports as he had learned to do in his graduate program, but the format, which didn't fit the current context, was not acceptable to other members of the staff. With little guidance from his colleagues Erik floundered almost desperately evening after evening, trying to figure out a format for presenting the data that would please the other staff members. Neither Robert nor I was familiar with social work or vocational evaluation forms, so we simply tried to wrestle with the problem alongside Erik, reading forms from his textbooks or examining various models he brought home from the library. Especially helpful was Robert's suggestion that Erik try to develop a "boilerplate"—a form that his colleagues would begin to recognize and count on and into which he could easily drop the data for each new client. There were countless trials and errors over the early months as Erik, with our questions and feedback, tried to develop a form that would meet the diverse and sometimes changeable interests of his supervisors and coworkers.

The oral presentations of his findings also produced considerable anxiety for Erik, for several reasons. He had come to expect implicit judgment from some of his colleagues, so simply anticipating a report made him nervous, and his nervousness tightened his physical body and constricted his mental processes. If someone questioned him about a recommendation, for example, he needed time to think and process his answer before responding. Without sufficient time to reflect, Erik could not always determine if a question was a statement conveying the idea that his judgment was being doubted or was instead a desire for information to support a judgment. The impatience of others sometimes led him to a hasty response that he later wished to reconsider. Certainly any of these anxieties might occur in any employee's first professional position, but the effects of Erik's head injury exacerbated their strength and compromised his ability to deal with them.

Despite these problems, during his two and a half years as a vocational counselor Erik developed greater awareness of himself. He learned to be more assertive by going directly to peers or supervisors about concerns or questions, and his empathy for the clients as well as for some of his fellow staff deepened. From his point of view, he derived the greatest personal satisfaction from applying for and receiving a contract from the Veterans' Administration to use the workshop as a vocational testing site. This contract would benefit the facility by generating new income. Erik initiated the proposal to his superiors and prepared the application, and when his institution received the contract Erik carried out the evaluations. While this additional work added pressure to his life, receiving the contract bolstered his self-esteem.

As parents, outside the situation, we could not always discern whether the working relationships were as highly charged and uncongenial as he described or whether he was overly sensitive. Frequently he reported that he felt like resigning. Usually those feelings subsided as he completed an evaluation that hung over his head or had some friendly interaction in the workplace. In times of discouragement we tried to help him use the conflict to investigate his own possible role in it or to learn something about himself and others from it. Though in hindsight we see that we may have encouraged him to stay too long in a situation that was at times more contentious than we understood, I know he gained competency in working with others and efficacy in making a contribution to society. For Erik, whose evolving sense of self depended on experimentation and mirroring or sometimes imitating others, the apparent shortage of improvisational flexibility at the sheltered workshop often deepened his isolation.

During the time Erik lived and worked in South Bend he became active in a local head injury support group. Although we had visited other such groups with him two or three times soon after his injury, he had strongly resisted regular participation. Initially he could not explain his resistance to such meetings; later he became vocal about not wanting to attend.

At the time, from 1985 until 1992, it was important for me to be around fully functioning people who could serve as models.

His words confirmed my suspicion that seeing his own needs reflected in others with different and sometimes more extreme impairments troubled and depressed him. By the time he achieved professional status as a rehabilitation counselor and began his job in South Bend, however, hc saw himself both as a person who had overcome a brain injury and as a professional committed to helping those with disabilities. In this support group Erik gave and received affirmation and satisfaction, and on occasion he interacted with statewide and regional head injury groups.

Not until I became more confident and competent in my own abilities did I feel able to help others in similar situations. I sort of wanted to operate on two levels: I wanted to relate professionally with parents and caregivers as well as empathetically to share the losses and struggles with the injured individuals.

Another essential way that Erik confronted loneliness and isolation was to seek out the Religious Society of Friends. From his Earlham days onward—in Lexington, Chicago, South Bend, and into his next move, to Bloomington, Indiana—he attached himself at least loosely to a Friends Meeting. His study and work schedules did not afford him much free time, but he found the weekly silent worship on First Days (Sundays) important to his identity and stability. In every meeting that we visited with him over the years we met gracious people who affirmed and cherished him. As he began to realize that his job as a vocational evaluator with its heavy load of paperwork that kept him working at home every evening and on the weekends beyond his regular eight-hour days was demanding too much from him, he used his family, some friends in the South Bend Friends Meeting, and the silence to consider alternative vocational directions. Out of these conversations and that waiting, he returned to consider again a library career. Library science seemed a desirable option: it would fulfill his desire to help others, his need to have an organized and orderly work environment that he could count on and contribute to, and his hope to have some time free from his job.

The difference between Erik's departures for college, Lexington, and Chicago and his leaving for Indiana University in Bloomington is striking. In all his previous trips we had helped him sort, select, and pack his belongings. Robert and he together had loaded the car or van carefully to get all the items safely in place. This time seemed no different at first as Robert and I helped Erik pack up his apartment and move things into our basement for storage. Two weeks later, however, Erik loaded his car and insisted on driving himself to Indiana University. Our concerns for his safety on a four-hour trip and his ability to locate a graduate housing complex on a large, unfamiliar university campus and unload at the end of the trip had more to do with other drivers' speed or impatience than with Erik's usually well-monitored driving. Despite our reservations of letting go yet another time, we sent him forth in hope that all would be well. Only a year later did we discover that, in fact, he had not traveled to Indiana University alone; a young woman friend had accompanied him. He had elected not to tell us at the time to avoid our advice and influence and to determine his own direction.

Although there was a kind of improvisational ebb and flow in Erik's relationship to his family and the world—out and then back, following closely the familiar and then leading outward to something unknown—between his college graduation and his decision to study library science, each motion contributed overall to the development of his ability to become the author of his own life story. Sometimes his movement, which seemed like self-direction to him, impressed us as impulsive or inadequately considered. To him our doubt-filled questions or cautionary advice felt controlling. When he broke off his long-distance relationship with his college girlfriend of six years, who was teaching in Korea, because he had met a female colleague at work who was very attractive to him, we regarded his actions as precipitous and impulsive, and we were candid and direct about our views.

As Erik's ideas about what he needed or wanted became stronger and more independent, we as parents had to confront several issues. When we were honest with ourselves we knew that we did not and could not know Erik's interior experience of anything, especially close personal relationships. We had to wrestle once again with the ways traumatic brain injury already had and would continue to affect the aspirations we had or the choices we might prefer for our son. As we worried about his vulnerability to being taken advantage of by others, we recognized the danger that our concerns could turn our fears for him into self-fulfilling prophecy. We also had to confront the consequences, often difficult to acknowledge and sometimes harder to negotiate, that arose from Erik's early dependence on us, his growing need for independence and self-direction, and what seemed to us to be a tendency for him to accept the wishes or directions of others in exchange for their acceptance. Such issues are the consequences of traumatic brain injury that, despite their subterranean life, bubble up to disturb day-to-day relationships—or to poison the underground waters of love on which all lives depend. When we persisted in expressing our judgments about what we thought to be appropriate or beneficial, we risked obstructing open communication and sometimes put Erik in a double bind with regard to his preferences. Increasingly Erik demonstrated ability to turn the tensions between his interests and ours to self-affirming ends.

This tension between your views and my desires that grew as I became more and more independent actually fueled my determination to recover to my fullest potential. To some extent, the differences in our viewpoints are common to all people. I decided somewhere along the way that I was going to live my life. My deep desire to live an independent life, not a dependent one, made it clear that at some point our paths needed to diverge. You know Robert Frost's poem: I took the road less traveled and that has made all the difference.

Over the years of Erik's continuing rehabilitation we have discovered that his life is not the only one under reconstruction. Indeed, the image of improvisation conveys the mutuality of this process. As he moved toward greater independence and confidence with a spirit of generosity, we often found ourselves clinging to memories of past dreams and weighed down with lingering grief. Although these two contradictory motions could not yield free-flowing and creative improvisations, Erik often appeared to use the tension between his forward-moving trust and our anxious concerns as a stable mooring against which to test himself further.

I have interpreted the improvisations of Erik's life during these post-injury years as a search for home, his home. In all his rehabilitation, academic study, social relationships, and employment he was rebuilding, perhaps restoring, the extended consciousness of his self house, what Damasio calls the autobiographical self. What is required fundamentally, according to Damasio, in the development of this self is stability and a boundary that the body provides. The reconstruction of Erik's self house depended on reorganizing the highly complex interactions of his brain, his emotions, and his musculoskeletal frame. His ability to come home to an altered self required him first to be located in his body. Only as Erik's brain could perceive and represent what was going on within his mind-body—his internal milieu—could he know himself as a "self" and relate to the constantly changing world around him.[6]

Throughout coma and beyond, the brain worked to restore its capacity to communicate dynamic representations within the body. With the return of consciousness Erik became aware of interactions with objects, people, and experiences in time and space that enlarged his autobiographical self. Memories returned and linked him to the past, and he could eventually imagine or project from the stability of his body-self (or self house) outward to others and forward to the future. To find his own uniqueness he also needed to establish ties to something greater than himself. Erik initially found these ties in his association with Friends and in the imagery of the Light or God within. Carl Jung describes this experience as the ego relating to the Self. The Sufi poet Kabir speaks of relationship within and between bodies with the metaphor of swinging:

Between the conscious and the unconscious,
the mind has put up a swing;
all earth creatures, even the supernovas, sway
    between these two trees,
and it never winds down.

Angels, animals, humans, insects by the million, also
    the wheeling sun and moon;
ages go by, and it goes on.
Everything is swinging: heaven, earth, water, fire,
and the secret one slowly growing a body.
Kabir saw that for fifteen seconds, and it made him a
    servant for life.[7]

Witnessing and participating in our son's efforts to reconstruct his
sense of self repeatedly left us swinging between the visible and the invisible. Robert and I visited Erik one Mother's Day weekend while he
was a student at the University of Kentucky, and together we went to
Pleasanthill, Kentucky, to see the restored Shaker community there. An
unanticipated and moving experience of our visit was the Louisville Ballet Company's performance of Doris Humphrey's *The Shakers*, choreographed in 1938. Sitting in the meeting house on backless plank benches,
we listened to the plaintive music and watched the precise choreogra-
phy, which depicted the physical response of worshipers to an inward
movement of the Spirit during an old Shaker meeting. Of the three of
us viewing the ballet performance from the benches that day, Erik
seemed paradoxically more ready or able figuratively to join the dance
through forgiveness, despite formidable impediments, while Robert and
I were still inclined to sit on the benches waiting and watching.

Accepting Vulnerability

All individuals and families   who suffer traumatic brain injury
must sooner   or later accept:
Brain injury   brings an end
to life   as they have known it.

As we stood on the springtime threshold of Erik's unfolding life in 1985, we had no hint that

What we call the beginning is often the end
And to make an end is to make a beginning.
The end is where we start from.[1]

Erik's loss of self through injury, unconsciousness, and confusion con-tributed to Robert's, Sonia's, and my loss of soul. Our sense of being in-tegrated body-mind-spirits participating in a benign and generative uni-verse was split asunder with Erik's accident. Sometimes in shock we felt like bodies whose minds had walked away; at other times our bodies ached without consolation from the spirit; occasionally, in fatigue and sympathetic identification with Erik, we experienced the diminishment of our cognitive functions. From the moment of crisis in May 1985 all we had with which to operate was what we knew, or thought we knew, about ourselves and our children, crippled or compromised as our understanding was by the intrusion of the unexpected. In our efforts to make a beginning from what was to us a tragic ending, we entered coma's silent region, picked up the pieces of our son and our ruptured trust and dreams, and moved into the realm of poetic language, where one learns to know his being through sounds, rhythm, signs, and symbols.[2] Here we attempted to make a beginning with the visible and invisible assistance of friends, family, and professionals. Erik's end, from which we and then he chose to make a beginning, led us on a long journey between ends and beginnings that has become over the years a continuous contest between attachment to old perceptions of the self and baffling new experiences of it, between control and relinquishment, between desire and love, and ultimately between an instrumental and a relational view of life.

Erik's experience of traumatic brain injury suddenly linked us to about 99,000 people in the United States who annually sustain traumatic brain injuries that result in lifelong disabilities. Marginalized by their injuries, this group is invisible to most Americans. Another 50,000 die from brain injuries, also unnoticed by society.[3] Chance events on one May Sunday afternoon pushed us out of the center of the human circle to the periphery, where we began to see life from the cultures of pain, disability, and death. Julia Kristeva, who studies the links between ethics and language, asserts that the question of ethics always arises whenever social codes or mores are "playfully shattered" to make room for something new—a need, desire, pleasure, or even negativity—to come forth.[4] I have concluded that brain injury presents a forced, not chosen, shattering not simply of mores and social contracts; it also shatters the self necessary for any social engagement or arrangement.

To put together the splintered pieces of the self and renegotiate the social contexts that previously sustained personality and identity requires poetic language. Because poetic language is concerned more with the material—sound and rhythms—than with rational reference or concepts, it recognizes that one who speaks may be divided between "unconscious and conscious motivations, that is, between physiological processes and social constraints."[5] With the aid of poetic language, which itself results from a kind of conversation between symbols (signs, syntax, and grammar) and the semiotic (instinctual drives and social and family constraints),[6] one may observe in the brain injured individual the rudimentary effort to recover one's sense of self through a dialectical language process. This process is played out first within the body and then between the individual's response to sound and rhythm and his or her effort to negotiate again the symbolic systems that facilitate communication. Traumatic brain injuries push the injured person, family members, and perhaps even entire societies into an experience more akin to free fall than to free play. All who are touched by brain injury indubitably require opening space for new ways of putting the self and its social relations together again—the opening that Kristeva describes. In this concluding chapter I seek to draw threads from the foregoing personal narrative into a larger social fabric in order to reflect on some ethical implications of brain injury for our understanding of the self and on the ways we live in society.

What Is Self?

From the first recognition that our son was critically injured with a traumatic brain injury, questions about selfhood dominated our attention. Prior to Erik's injury I thought of the self largely in psychological terms as a closed and relatively stable entity, much as I did characters in drama or works of fiction. Though as a parent of developing children and a teacher of literary texts I knew that environmental factors contribute to or impede an individual's growth, I considered much of that development to be guided by the internal operations of each self. Carl Jung's theories of consciousness, particularly a collective unconscious that shapes people through image and archetype across time and space, had influenced me, so I did acknowledge some potential interplay between selves certainly within and even beyond the primary social unit of the family or culture. Traumatic brain injury pushed me further away than feminism already had from traditional or modernist philosophical categories toward provisional interpretations of self and social relations.

Erik's brain injury turned what had simply been an interesting academic debate about essentialism and contingency into a matter of extreme personal significance. In the absence of consciousness and physical responsiveness, is there a self? If so, where is it? What constitutes it? At the bleakest moments Erik seemed to have no essence, and he was surely not able to invent or reinvent himself in discernible ways. As we listened to medical personnel talk to Erik and discuss his condition with us, I also wondered "who" they had in mind when they spoke. He could not be to them our special first-born child; more likely he was a physical being, described in case notes, who presented a familiar collection of symptoms that made him part of a group labeled "brain injured," a status against which they could measure his progress toward or regression from "selfhood."

As we witnessed Erik's physical, emotional, and cognitive changes during the early weeks and months following injury, two perceptions of selfhood as I had formerly conceived it changed. First, I realized that selfhood did not lodge largely in what we loosely call the mind or psyche, but resided instead at the cellular, chemical, and neural levels of a human being. Gradually I recognized that there was an exquisite, if disturbed and disheveled, communication occurring in the body-brain of Erik. Without that he could never be again a "self." Second, our persistent interactions with him and the effect those seemed to have on his awakening and heightening awareness confirmed the self's dependence on others and its responsiveness to narration. Experientially I discerned some evidence that "the mind has put up a swing between the conscious and the unconscious . . . and it never winds down" and that all living forms—animals, plants, stars, moon, and sun—partake of this movement. Acknowledgment of this intricate communication system within an individual organism and between human organisms required me to entertain the possibility that the human brain is in some ways a story-making organ.

From such observations and reflections I concluded that the human being is neither essentialist nor purely contingent, but both. Without boundaries and a stable internal system—what one might consider a physical essence—there could be no knowing being. Without *permeable* boundaries through which inter-being communication can occur there would be no species community or society. Such thoughts first made it impossible for me to assume that Erik would or could be restored simply by medical interventions. Then my growing awareness of our human dependence on one another's contributions to our selfhood filled me with awe. Every interaction with Erik, every conversation with him that I experienced or observed, every emotional outburst that we mediated became a source of wonder and investigation.

Erik's injury also made transparent the reality that the consequences of traumatic brain injuries are not confined to the injured individual, despite the fact that our medical, rehabilitation, and educational institutions focus their interventions on the injured individual and usually encourage family members to leave the care of their loved one to the professionals. Even in those cases where families do rely totally on medical or rehabilitation institutions, eventually a time comes when the family member can no longer remain a patient and must return to a former home, find a new place to reside, or be moved to a long-term care facility. In any of these cases, the family itself is pulled into the open, unmarked space that traumatic brain injury has created and then must adapt to the needs of their beloved and adjust their own personal and professional lives to accommodate those needs financially, emotionally, and physically.

If one previously thought of her or his own self as a relatively stable life set on a clear, progressive trajectory, brain injury to a member of the family radically challenges that notion. Because mothers are still regarded by their families, employers, and societies—and by themselves—as the primary nurturers of their families, they often bear the heaviest responsibility for adaptations. In two-parent families this usually means that the father's career or employment will remain on track; if the mother was employed outside the home she may, in order to assume the responsibilities previously handled by medical or rehabilitation professionals, reduce her hours or her professional productivity, both of which will jeopardize her own employment benefits, her professional opportunities, and her self-perception. Over time both the primary care provider and the injured family member will become invisible to the larger society, for the provider has quietly picked up the social obligation. The stress that traumatic brain injury places on families often fragments the family. The Brain Injury Association reports that the incidence of divorce in marriages where one spouse has suffered a traumatic brain injury is 80 percent.

In single-parent homes, or in cases where the injured member is a parent, the demands on the sole parent or other siblings are compounded immeasurably. Often the injured family member will be left alone with a television set for extended periods. As I write, a single mother in New Zealand has won a precedent-setting legal case against such invisibility. Recognizing the unjust financial, not to mention physical and psychic, burden placed on the family for the prolonged and intensive medical and rehabilitative care of her severely injured son, the courts awarded her a financial settlement that will support her son's lifelong needs. Brain injury raises profound questions about the adequacy of the nuclear family's attempts to sustain alone a life-giving web of relationships necessary for self-reconstruction.

For siblings or children of brain-injured family members, caution or fear of the unexpected often replaces trust. Siblings, children, and parents also often struggle with guilt for not having to deal with the deficits of injury themselves and thus find it harder to carry out their own goals or aspirations. Spouses or parents of injured loved ones may begin to exhibit their own difficulties in concentration or memory that can result from intense identification with the injured family member or simply from strain and fatigue. The prolonged demands of care for the injured person and of adjustments required of the rest of the family often bring latent unresolved interpersonal issues to the surface or generate hostilities that ultimately dissolve family bonds, including those of marriage. All these effects are intensified in conditions of economic poverty or where reliable social networks and educational resources are limited. In short, because brain injury to anyone in a family system threatens everyone's static views of selfhood, some form of narrative therapy— opportunities to tell the story of the impact of this experience from as many angles as possible—seems absolutely necessary to the reconstruction process of everyone involved.

Although it is impossible to assess the personal views of selfhood held by individual doctors, nurses, therapists, or teachers who worked with Erik in crisis and during the years beyond, my experience is that personal views are always subsumed under professional protocols. The reliance on medical technologies to save lives or rehabilitation strategies to make patients functional again places the medical professional or rehabilitation therapist at the center of attention, often focusing more on the assistance offered than on the patient as a whole being. Paradoxically, the patient may be instrumentalized—a mere object to fit into schedules and protocols—as he or she proves the efficacy of the technological intervention or the rehabilitation strategy. When the patient reaches viability in the trauma unit, or much later achieves the fundamental goals of rehabilitation, for example, he or she is passed on to another department or to someone else.

As Erik moved through the various medical and rehabilitation systems, no professionals followed his progress or kept track of what interventions had worked most effectively. Surely this pattern suggests a reductionist approach to selfhood, for each profession contributes its discrete specialty to the reconstruction process. But the highly compartmentalized nature of this approach, plus the fact that the patient is generally separated from his former social context during this passage, leaves the task of personal integration and the more subtle work of meaning-making largely unaddressed. As I look still further underneath this pattern of treatment, recognizing that often it is not the patient but the professionals and their protocols that are affirmed in the struggle for survival, I find lurking a fairly mechanistic view of the self whose worth is calculable in economic costs.

Control and Surrender

As has become amply clear in the preceding chapters, traumatic brain injury brings an abrupt end to any real control, or the illusion of it, that one has over her own or her loved ones' lives. While he was comatose Erik was not only apparently far beyond our discernible reach but also totally dependent on the expertise of people whom we didn't know and who didn't know us. With the exception of two hours each twenty-four-hour period for the first three weeks, we had to relinquish our vulnerable son to the care of those unknown. This absence of control to protect, to care for, or even to try to rescue endured. Sometimes our powerlessness battled brutally with our determination to influence—what others might have regarded as control—the quality of care Erik received and to affect its outcome.

Through every stage and change this struggle between control and surrender persisted. It continued internally for us as parents even when Erik left for college and we were no longer in physical proximity. Because we chose from the outset to stay involved with Erik, we became attuned to his needs and vulnerabilities, we recognized signals that others who saw him intermittently could not detect, and we gradually discerned the implications of his injury and experimented with him on ways to compensate for losses or impairments. Because we could foresee potential problems, we were inclined to protect against them or ward them off. This level of investment and commitment could not be sustained over time, especially as Erik's desire for independence grew.

We experienced this desire to control in relation not only to Erik but also to our daughter, Sonia, and our own lives. When all foundations are shaken one seeks ways to hang on lest one lose her moorings altogether. As Sonia became a teenager she had to cope with typical parental control issues that had been exacerbated by the terror of an automobile crash that resulted in traumatic brain injury.

The urge to control is of course not limited to anxious parents. It runs throughout most medical and rehabilitation institutions, educational systems, insurance companies, and legal institutions with some puzzling, even pernicious, variations. For example, limiting our access to Erik to two out of every twenty-four hours when he was in the trauma unit protected the control of medical personnel. While it is eminently reasonable not to have entire families underfoot impeding medical services in acute care situations, often decisions to restrict the presence of family members are made principally for the ease and secrecy of the medical professional without consideration of a family member's potential usefulness to the patient's healing. The pernicious side of the need to control shows itself when anyone suggests that the presence of another person threatens to alter the quality of a professional's services. Such suggestions imply that if a family member will not bow to the required control, then the professional will have to relinquish his or her responsibility to give the best care possible. Within families control is often maintained with threats to remove approval or love. Here one begins to see the ways intimidation supports control and always disempowers those who often need most to be empowered.

Over the years I came to understand that the struggle between control and surrender is fundamentally a spiritual contest contrived by the ego to test its own limits and to extend its influence over the universe and others in it. The urge to control is always driven by the controller's perceptions, preferences, or will and is aimed at making other people or situations conform to the controller's ideas or values. When one confronts the random or the uncontrollable in life one must either crumble before it or relinquish. We experienced our share of crumbling and despair, which left me feeling powerless. By contrast, relinquishment appeared to be a choice that inexplicably opened and deepened my care for Erik and my sense of power to assist without demanding anything in return.

During our months in hospitals and subsequently in educational institutions we met many professionals who daily gave their skills of care without demanding control. Whenever this occurred we as family and they as professionals entered a cooperative relationship that opened a much wider healing space for Erik, not to mention ourselves.

Dancing with Desire and Love

Surrender is to love as desire may be to control. Whereas letting go opens a channel through which love can flow, desire attaches us to those objects we desire and inclines us toward control for its fulfillment. Throughout our participation in Erik's self-reconstruction, in our observations in hospitals, and in our conversations with other individuals with brain injuries and their families, desire and love emerged repeatedly as strong and necessary, though often competing, forces in a family's life following traumatic brain injury. We experienced the whole range of emotions associated with the term *desire:* sometimes we felt it as profound yearning for that which no longer existed; often we expressed desire through our will not to give up on Erik; occasionally, especially when I saw agile, mentally flexible young people having fun together, I felt desire as covetousness rush through me; every now and then desire drew close to love in its purity of intention for our son's well-being. I have come to distinguish desire from love, however, through my own personal wrestling with these closely related impulses and the consequences each produced in me. No one affixed these terms to our struggles in the throes of crisis, but from the perspective of more than a dozen years I can see that the choices that confronted us every morning upon waking until lying down at night fell either toward desire or tipped toward love. Sometimes desire and love danced together tensely.

Every family who receives word that a loved one has sustained a traumatic brain injury wishes with every ounce of available energy that the injury would not have occurred. Desire for preferred outcomes drives the repetitious recital of "what ifs." What if he hadn't gone on the outing? What if he had not changed cars? Each family has its own recital of such questions: What if she had let me take her poems to the post office? What if he had left the office at his usual time? Then, with the protective assistance of the psychological defense called denial, families of the brain injured find themselves deeply attached to the images and memories imprinted in their minds of their loved ones as they have always known them. Our abiding desire for many weeks and months, which stretched feebly into years, was that our child would again be who and what we thought he was. Despite the realism of trauma unit physicians and nurses—an attitude that families experience as extreme pessimism—extended families and the general population encourage such desires by always inquiring if an injured member is getting back to 100 percent or "normal." Indeed, to let go of this basic desire for full recovery from traumatic brain injury seems tantamount to abandoning one's loved one, so most families and the injured themselves, when they can, cling to it desperately.

In the clutches of desire I experienced or witnessed over and over the temptation to blame someone or something for what had happened. As humans filled with the desire to know or to understand—in short, to control—we cannot easily accept the inexplicable, the random, the unexpected. Though initially the injured person usually receives compassion or sympathy from family and friends, as the severity and uncertainty of the outcome settle in, they may begin to blame the injured person himself or herself. In the trauma unit we heard one mother railing against her comatose daughter for not waking up, for putting her parents through so much agony, for not wanting to help herself. God is also frequently charged with allowing this devastation to occur. And often, in quite convoluted efforts to make meaning of random events, loved ones interpret the events to be acts of God or God's will.

It is a short step from the temptation, born of desire, to blame God or unseen forces for an injury to the temptation to bargain for results that we want. Bargaining from our attachment to our injured child or spouse or parent whose continuation in that image and form seems essential for our own identity, occurs both simply and with nuanced sophistication. In anguished intercessory prayer one pleads simply from desire, requesting "if this" and promising "then we'll do that." As enduring consequences of an injury become more apparent, bargaining may turn more complex as one tries every therapeutic intervention, always seeking the desired outcome, or begins to play differing rehabilitation approaches against one another. When Erik could say a few words and recognize us, I recall feeling that if he were to plateau at that point that would be enough, even if he were bedfast. But as I grew accustomed to his rudimentary speech forms I began bargaining, as in longing, for more. If only he could walk unsupported. Then, if only he could run. Then, if only he could play basketball. Go to school. Get married.

Driven by desire, the families of the injured and the injured themselves, when they are cognitively aware, always struggle with the temptation to deny losses or impairments. Even therapists, medical doctors, psychologists, and social workers, who consider it their responsibility to help the patient accept new realities, may be equally strongly driven by desire to disabuse the patient of baseless hope, thereby further increasing the patient's resistant denial. I watched Erik intently labor over math problems that he had previously handled with grace, denying the changes that had taken place. Several years after Erik's injury I met another fine young man—an aspiring poet before his injury during his first year of college—trying desperately to make a poem again. I stood beside him in his room, watching him press the print command on his computer. When the page appeared, a little wrinkled, he handed it to me proudly. "Do you want to read my poem?" On the page were broken phrases, words that to me seemed random, but in the spaces between the words lay the lost poet and his desire, laced with denial.

The relationship among desire, denial, and motivation in the service of, or as an expression of, the self is exceedingly complex. Erik's desire to do advanced mathematics or the young poet's desire to arrange sounds and rhythm into poems may have held off resignation and despair and eventually motivated them to find new interests. Their desires may have enabled them to resist or deny invisibility or non-beingness. The urge for individuality or autonomy in Western cultures is always driven by desire that ironically is mediated not as much as we like to believe by individual choice but by imitation of an other, a standard, a hero, or an idealized image. Desire permits us to believe that we are developing or protecting our own rights to be ourselves, to distinguish ourselves from others, while in fact we become deeply attached to that which objectively or subjectively represents autonomy or individuality for us.

Brain injury exposes desire's attachment to the illusion of the autonomous self in at least two ways. First, although it took us a while to recognize this fully, the brain injured are utterly dependent on interaction with and imitation of others. Lacking the capacity for guile, they unashamedly imitate in small and grand ways those behaviors, attitudes, or people who presumably represent something of value to them. Second, working with Erik over the years opened a window on the ways we, the uninjured in the general population, conduct our own lives. I began to notice the imitative qualities in all human exchanges, from the most mindless acts, to highly sophisticated discussions, to geopolitical decisions. In those of us without brain injuries the capacity for self-deceit and defense has not been impaired, so we continue to operate our lives largely through our desires, which paradoxically often lead us less toward freedom than toward bondage to our attachments.

I give so much attention to desire because as a parent of a child who struggled to cope with a brain injury I recognized that my desires—and much later Erik's own desires—were invariably tinged, if not filled, with fear that they might not be realized; hence my attitudes and actions became preservational and protective. On the surface our family desires for Erik's restoration looked optimistic and filled with hope, yet they were always tied to a memory image or a projection of some ideal we wished for him and for ourselves that lay beyond the present moment and present reality. Desire can deaden or diminish our experience of our own and others' being and of the world.

Even many medical and rehabilitation practices, most of our educational programs, and managed health care systems are developed and governed by the play of desire. To preserve or restore health or to contribute to the intellectual formation and social responsibility of individuals, professionals in these fields create procedures or set standards by which to measure progress toward the desired objective, whether of cure, functionality, or independence. The protocols and procedures, the regimens and tests, provide parameters within which each patient or student performs and defines himself. When, however, such systems become rigid and offer little flexible space for experimentation, for deviation, or for heterogeneity, they may unintentionally narrow the options, restrict aspirations, and undermine the capacity for establishing associative bonds beyond one's own kind, class, or condition.

The influence of managed health care systems, themselves driven by desire for profits, compounds the vulnerability of the injured by limiting time for or access to rehabilitation therapies. During the fifteen years since Erik's injury research on the human brain has yielded significant information about the brain's plasticity and even its regenerative capacities, but, paradoxically, the amount of time head-injured patients may spend in rehabilitation facilities to receive intensive therapeutic interventions has decreased dramatically. During a 1998 return visit to the Alfred I. Dupont Hospital for Children I learned that residential rehabilitation time for a brain-injured patient had dropped over the fifteen-year period from up to six months to six to eight weeks. The press first to move families out of the hospital and then to get patients out of the hospitals and back into their homes with insufficient support often leaves these patients isolated by physical impairments that prohibit their mobility or by a lack of stimulating interactions. Without training, most families are ill equipped to provide the sustained care that is required to deal successfully with the emotional, physical, and cognitive needs of a family member with brain injury.

Despite the tremendous instinctual sway of desire and its useful, preservational aspect, it always holds the desirer captive to that for which he or she longs. Although the energy of desire is strong and may even be turned away from oneself or transformed, it alone is inadequate for bringing individual being—personality—into relationship with Being, which animates all physical and mental-spiritual life. Erik's desire, even accompanied by Herculean efforts, to be again a facile mathematics student left him feeling divided inside himself and isolated from others. Over time the creative energy of love extended unconditionally to him and by himself toward himself opened a space for the fearsome and the ambiguous and the bizarre—for his strangeness to himself—and enabled him to find his being through poetic language and story. Language and the capacity to communicate became for Erik what Martin Heidegger called "the house of being." Poetic language released him to be a speaking subject, to express his subjectivity, and to know himself through dialogue and relationship with other beings. Love that frees one to care for or to act on the behalf of another, even for the self as an other, without an expectation of returns or specified outcomes establishes ties between being and Being within the solitary individual and among human beings within the human circle.

Ethical Implications: From Justice to Answerability

Love, as I refer to it, contains ontological, religious, ethical, physical, biological, and psychological aspects, all of which Robert and I experienced as participant-observers of Erik's self-reconstruction. Love's importance to individuals coping with traumatic brain injury is indisputable; its relevance for examining the ethical implications of traumatic brain injury may be less obvious. Etymologically, *ethics* comes from *ethos*, which denotes a person's characteristic and distinguishing attitudes, and thus is closely tied to our notions of the self. Traumatic brain injury presents a unique ethical dilemma because, striking at the center of an individual's viability, it threatens to annihilate the self. Even before we grasped the extent of Erik's injuries, our assumptions that we were entitled to and would receive justice were seriously undermined. There is never any justice associated with the disintegration and suffering caused by traumatic brain injury. Furthermore, by breaking apart a self and releasing into our midst the aberrant, the bizarre, and the amnesiac, severe brain injury challenges many of the social codes and mores that govern human interaction. Brain injury brings with it resentment and regret as well as the yearning for pleasure and the satisfaction of desire for which there is no ameliorating response of justice. Where, we wondered, in our conceptions of justice, whether shaped by utilitarian or Judeo-Christian values, is there the social space needed for those afflicted by brain injury to wail in confusion, to experiment, or to attempt a reconstruction of their being-house in broken poetic language? How can we incorporate the brain injured into our lives and let them teach us with their gestures, signs, and halting language?

Without justice as a guide for answering pressing, messy questions such as these, we starkly faced a choice between life and death in relating to Erik. To leave him in coma's silence, in his agitation, or at any subsequent stage of his journey would have been to reject life and relationship. Though for us the rudder of justice had been destroyed by the accident, health care providers around us nevertheless sought to treat Erik and other critically injured patients fairly, using technological ingenuity to save people who previously would have died from their injuries. For health professionals and many psychologists and educators, to treat the injured justly means providing intensive acute and rehabilitative care of fixed duration; it may mean offering worker's compensation or Medicaid; it could include placing an injured individual in an assisted residential program. Essential as these early-stage medical and rehabilitative interventions are, even they can be severely limited by what a managed care contract stipulates or can rapidly diminish if the patient has no insurance. Furthermore, all such efforts alone cannot provide the individualized care and attention required, over a longer rather than shorter time, for the unpredictable, intricate, and complex process of reconstructing the self.

Ethics based on justice has a long and rich tradition in most Western cultures, and the contributions to our collective welfare that are derived from public decisions informed by standards of justice should not be undervalued. Betrayals of justice abound, however, especially for the poor and otherwise marginalized. Traumatic brain injuries enforce marginalization *in extremis* and present two unique obstacles to the instrumentalist orientation of decisions based on justice. Even accepting some basic similarities in traumatic brain injuries, beyond the most rudimentary comparisons no two injuries will be alike and no two patients will respond alike to similar injuries or treatments. Furthermore, because the long-range consequences from such injuries are nearly always uncertain, it is difficult to prescribe approaches on the basis of predictable or reliable outcomes. Whether selected therapeutic means guarantee a desired, utilitarian outcome can never be definitively ascertained. In the face of such ambiguities, those with brain injuries are usually assisted intensively for a few months to a year and then left to manage as best they can.

Precisely because traumatic brain injuries afflict such individual consequences, attempting to make ethical decisions about treatment on the basis of principles of justice such as rights and equity seems impossible. From our personal decision to stay aggressively engaged with Erik through every stage, and from the generous attention Erik received from a host of people, the ground of our ethical thinking radically shifted from justice to care to answerability, carrying me to the heart of ethics: the self and its need for care and to care. Choosing to companion Erik—to break the bread of loss and pain with him—focused our attention increasingly on the mystery of our vulnerable son's struggle and needs and on imagining ways to respond to those.

The impulse to care, which arose instinctively in us as parents, depends on the affective basis of existence and differs fundamentally from ethical approaches that are rooted in law and principle. Nel Noddings explains in *Caring: A Feminine Approach to Ethics and Moral Education* that caring as an ethical approach implies a kind of reciprocity different from "that of 'contract' theorists such as Plato and John Rawls." She argues compellingly that "it is our longing for caring—to be in that special relation—that provides the motivation for us to be moral." In contrast, ethics of principle, which promote universalizability, always see aberrant behavior as exceptional, separate us from each other, and tempt us to self-righteousness when others do not adhere to our revered principle.[7] The limits of ethics based on justice that Noddings describes are graphically clear in cases of traumatic brain injury, for without consciousness, temporarily bereft of familiar social context, and lacking language and storying capacity, the injured individual cannot contractually exchange anything and falls outside the norm of human interaction.

We as family were not alone in choosing compassion, or care, over justice. Based purely on the principles of justice or equity, there was no need for Princeton Day School to take Erik back into its community. Guided by justice he would have followed the advice of several professionals and entered a special education classroom in a public school. Ethical choices based on care, however, begin in effect where justice leaves off,[8] inviting us to consider our need to care in relation to individual needs and interests, differing abilities, and the associative and spiritual requirements of the injured. The challenge of reassembling a shattered self, rudely forced upon individuals, families, social institutions, and the social space, called us to reevaluate all our moral assumptions.

An ethics of care moves beyond justice by its double focus on the injured person as an end in himself or herself and on the human answerability of the ones who care. Though the first part—seeing the injured always as an end—may be hard to maintain when consciousness is absent or when strange, even dangerous, behaviors are expressed, the concept of answerability may provide an even more formidable challenge to our understanding. Paradoxically, our severely injured son taught me about answerability not as an abstraction but, through his years of reshaping his life in response to what had occurred to him, as a reality. Erik and I never discussed answerability. I witnessed it and only much later, as I wrote this book, attached a term to what I have experienced. To make it clear, I turn to literature for assistance.

Within a story within his story within Dostoevsky's novel *The Brothers Karamazov,* Father Zosima tells Alyosha of Zosima's young brother Markel's reflections as he lay close to death. Speaking to his mother, Markel says, "My own dear blood, my sweet joy, know that this is the truth and that every one of us is answerable for everyone else and for everything. I don't know how to explain it to you, but I feel it so strongly that it hurts."[9] For Markel, answerability seems to be a tangible, physical experience, registered in his body, that altered his whole orientation toward his own life and world. Given his weakened state one might reasonably assume that to be answerable could not mean, as we commonly think, that he should take control over events or direct others' decisions. Whereas we think of being answerable as taking responsibility for someone else's action or need, through Zosima's story Dostoevsky defines answerability as each person's obligation first to imagine what another is going through and then to answer, with his or her own life, for what he or she has experienced, so that what has been witnessed and understood will not remain ineffectual.[10] To be answerable for another compels one to acknowledge and to respond to one's own experience. Using one's own life to make visible or more bearable—to call forth—another person's experience is fundamentally creative. It requires an assent to freedom—freedom to experiment, to let go, to stand in relation to the past and future differently, to be willing to open one's self to possibility and change. In order to imagine the life of another one must recognize a living dialogue within oneself between an *I* as subject and a *you* necessary for communication and action. Just as the artist who writes a novel seeks to express a unity between the work of art and life, so each of us, to be answerable "for everyone else and everything," must make from our lives a work of art that embodies, in open service or sacrifice, what we have experienced and understood. Answerability permits us to stand in relation to ourselves and others expectantly, but without expectation. It cleans the windows of perception, making visible our intersubjectivity and leading toward reconciling ourselves to that which we have rejected in ourselves or to those who have been maimed or marginalized in our communities.

No one, neither the doctors nor we as Erik's parents, could be responsible for Erik in the ways we generally think of taking responsibility for others. He ultimately had to walk the circuitous path that follows traumatic brain injury himself. Indeed, he has been answerable to his experience. Yet he was not left utterly alone because numerous others chose, even if not deliberately, to demonstrate their own answerability. In attending to the care of Sonia, in rigging up an old television and VCR for a thirteenth birthday party, in recording classical guitar music or the Bach Brandenburg concertos for us to play for Erik, Pat and Mike were answerable. Medical and rehabilitation professionals who offered their understanding as well as skill were answerable. Erik's school advisor, who became an interpreter of Erik's condition for students and faculty, was answerable. Teachers and administrators who pushed the limits of their own backgrounds and understanding to elicit from Erik what lay scrambled inside modeled answerability as the heart of an ethics of care. Erik's small circle of friends who chose to stand by him risked answerability. Fred and Winnie Hoover, who simply opened their home for three months to a family of strangers and said, "Be at home," were answerable. And so were many who merely waited at a distance in reverent love and hope. To be answerable does not even require visibility. One year after Erik's injury I received a short, clear note from a Friend whom I believe we had not seen during that year. In it he said he was giving what he could by performing twice-daily intercessory meditations for Erik. That too was being answerable "for everyone and everything."

After reading this book in manuscript, Dr. Macellari made the concept of answerability transparent. Because he had patiently and steadfastly assisted Erik in returning again and again to issues resulting from the accident until they were resolved, Dr. Macellari companioned Erik into independence and capability. Now, several years after they had worked together, he said, "The accomplishments Erik has achieved after all he has gone through is nothing short of miraculous." Through his own professional life and example, Dr. Macellari has been answerable not simply for Erik. After fifteen years his words reminded me how far Erik has traveled on this journey and confirmed the power of answerability.

As I sat in hospital corridors, watching some children linger in coma or wither idly without active interaction, waiting for our own child and others' children as they struggled to reclaim a moderately stable gait or to follow three-step directions, lamenting with other parents the loss of dreams that are always deposited with our seeds in our children, and continuing to listen in the silences and to see dimly into the dark for hints about how a human being becomes a self a second time, two things happened to me. As the foregoing narrative demonstrates, I slowly perceived that traumatic brain injury provides the grossest opening through which to examine how any of us becomes and continues to sustain a self. Through all our interactions with Erik, I also learned that within our own bodies, through our gestures, our thoughts, our words, and our acts, we call into being or cut off our own and others' selfhood.

Such discoveries have compelled me to look closely at the meaning we make of illness, injury, and disability in a society that chases health, longevity, and invincibility. What kind of tables are we setting in our personal and social houses? Who will be welcome at these tables, and who will be excluded? Writing movingly about family life with a son born with Down syndrome, Michael Bérubé addresses these and related questions, concluding persuasively that as humans we share a common characteristic: "the desire to communicate, to understand, to put ourselves in some mutual, reciprocal form of contact with one another."[11] In this desire for reciprocal communication lies our hope and the means for resetting our tables, enlarging the numbers who may sit there, and appreciating the diversity of those who come for nourishment.

Although I share faith with Bérubé in Habermas's theory of "communicative action"—the notion that an ideal society "resembles an 'ideal speech situation' in which all conversants speak freely in an atmosphere free of domination, coercion, or power asymmetry of any kind"[12]—traumatic brain injury has taught me a second indispensable lesson. When our fellow human beings are deprived of consciousness and language, for either short or enduring periods of time, we with consciousness, language, and conscience must listen and speak on their behalf. If we walk into the terrain opened by traumatic brain injury personally with another or merely with empathetic imagination, we will confront our true condition of vulnerability and have the opportunity to consider how to live ethically with one another in that condition.

Vulnerability: Opening Sacred Space

An ethics of care rests on vulnerability and answerability. Traumatic brain injury makes vulnerability visible and creates an imperative need to put together the smashed pieces of an individual's life as well as to incorporate the experience into our collective social and psychic life. If we accept vulnerability and choose to be answerable in the face of the fortuitous and the disintegrating, we may open a space that becomes holy because it offers the injured and uninjured together the flexible room and the raw materials with which to reconstruct a house of being. In such a space diminishment and loss, confusing or repetitive speech, frustration, endless repetition, and aberrant behavior become these raw materials. All such houses are built with poetic language, language that is imprinted in the body and animated by the senses, exchanged through verbal symbols between bodies and minds, and extended into cultures. The reconstruction occurs on several levels simultaneously: within the body-brain system, between the injured and the non-injured who have ventured into the terrain of brain injury, and within and among all social institutions on which every self depends. When any facet of this multileveled interaction is ignored or obstructed we expose the dubious nature of the notion that the self is a closed subjective entity. Those who accept this faulty assumption abandon those with brain injuries, pressing them to the farthest fringes of society by leaving them alone or placing them in small homogeneous groups.

As the foregoing narrative implies, Erik's sense of self was not the only reconstruction required by the accident; it also forced us, as mother, father, and sister, to redefine our understandings of ourselves and to reshape our relationships to one another and to the world. It is instructive to note the reconstructions the three of us have fashioned in attempting to answer the call to care, despite our similar yet distinct vulnerabilities.

As I neared the completion of this manuscript, Sonia asked me why I had written it. Stepping outside the role of observer-narrator, I answered as her mother.

Throughout much of my life writing has been my way of navigating my interior and the external worlds. Initially, after Erik's accident, writing offered me a way to "hang on" when destruction and chaos threatened to overtake me. In the bleakest hours I wrote to reach Erik, who was lost to me in a dark realm I could not fathom. I wrote, as it were, to call to him. Then as days led into months, writing served all of the following functions, sometimes sequentially and sometimes simultaneously. I wrote to hold darkness at bay and to grope toward some ray of light. A little later writing became a chronicle, a means of remembering terms in the new medical and rehabilitation languages I was learning and of recording significant events in Erik's journey. I wrote to interpret Erik's condition to his friends and to family. During his high school years I wrote to advocate on his behalf, and now that he speaks ably for himself, I write so that others may appreciate the intricacies of the being we call the self. Throughout this process my pen has moved back and forth between risk and protection.

In the end, this experience has required me to confront personal and cultural myths that die hard because they have indelibly imprinted my life. Myths that honor the heroic, the powerful, the orderly, the continuous and progressive, the brilliant, and the beautiful leave little room for the unexpected, for the discontinuous, and for weakness. I see more clearly now how such myths undermine relational being by encouraging competition and narcissistic perfectionism. My early hope that "perfection" would kiss our son and restore him in my image has, thankfully, been radically revised. Through Erik's restorying of his life and my written searching, I have been written toward a broader understanding of perfection. To be perfect is to accept our vulnerability, to be open to change, and to risk everything on the unfinished self, the self always being called forth.

Looking through Robert's eyes, and from conversations with other fathers of children who have suffered serious brain injuries, I have learned how deep the identification is between fathers and sons. So pervasive is our human faith in the continuity of generations that when it is threatened or thrown into question a profound reordering of one's values is necessary. Robert's paternal instinct for sacrifice was so strong that if he could have crawled into Erik's bed and Erik could have walked away energetic and healthy, he would have happily made the exchange. He writes:

From the moment of the accident to the present day, I have lived under inescapable clouds of grief, fear, and anger. Although I seldom express these emotions directly, they live within me. I struggle against them day by day. The accident changed our lives forever, cut lasting scars, and even now requires adjustments that are difficult to accept. Of course the pain today takes a form different from that of fifteen years ago. Now it arises from relinquishing dreams that will not be realized and from seeing hardships frequently placed in Erik's and our paths that would not have been there without the accident.

My difficulties in adjusting to the accident have given me a new understanding of what it means to walk through the valley of the shadow of death. We walk that valley not only at a moment of crisis but also as the shadows from the crisis lengthen throughout the remainder of our lives. I have tried to accept the unwanted realities in our family's life and to forgive those responsible for the accident in which our innocent son was nearly killed and suffered grievous injuries. Yet my religious faith, counseling, and repeated efforts over fifteen years have not closed the festering wound in my heart and soul. I still feel unspeakable sadness about the continuing consequences of the accident, and I struggle against the recurring anxiety that evil and suffering may strike at any moment.

The aching wounds opened by our son's injuries also have led me to understand some fundamental truths about myself and about life. For example, I now know the wisdom of living in the present moment and of appreciating what I have when I have it. Whereas before the accident I was always looking ahead to the intensely anticipated future achievements of Erik and Sonia, now I appreciate them in the present for the wonderful individuals that they are. I also learned that high achievement is not the highest value in life, unless by "achievement" we mean giving one's utmost to loving God and to laying down our lives for others. I am learning to listen more sensitively, to be less judgmental, to be more patient, and to accept that which I cannot change.

I also take great joy in Erik's miraculous recovery, and in the many fine qualities he radiates, particularly his compassion, his forgiveness, his tolerance, his determination, his industriousness, his insight, his thoughtfulness, and his integrity. No one could wish for a finer son. I am constantly uplifted by his greatest gift to me: his love for and acceptance of me despite my weaknesses and difficulties in letting go of frozen expectations.

The injury to our son also led me to vow never to hurt another parent's child. If, without suffering an accident, everyone would make that promise, then prejudice, poverty, wars, and inhumanities would cease.

Many times I have felt that the heart-breaking burdens were too much to bear. But, miraculously, I also have known that it would make no sense to jeopardize my relationships with Ruthann and Sonia and Erik or to throw my own life away because of a dysfunctionality that could arise from negative thoughts and painful emotions. That unshakable conviction, which other people who suffer can also share, has always been enough to keep up the good struggle.

To parents invested in continuity, sacrifice and looking backward seem natural inclinations when the possibility of seeing parental hopes fulfilled by one's offspring is challenged. Paradoxically, siblings who do not project their own continuity through one another are better equipped to redefine the future and to live flexibly as they grow into it. Sonia, who at thirteen penned faithfully in her 1985 diary "keep praying," hints at twenty-eight of the importance of answerability to the injured and uninjured alike.

The accident remains a life-defining event for me; Erik's need and his life made everything I did matter. The accident marks time for me. I understand myself differently before and after it. Because it occurred when I was "coming of age," it brought a wrenching loss of innocence, perhaps a fall from grace.

Because the accident happened at such a formative period in my life, I realize that it has impacted me in a very different way from my parents. They had lived a much larger portion of their lives before the accident, whereas I am living the larger portion of my life after it. Erik, and my relationship to him as a big brother, was a central part of my world construction, which was completely changed one Sunday afternoon. In an instant my world was dismantled and my experiences of loss, love, fear, grief, and hope became both blessing and curse. To have too much hope leaves little room for grief; to grieve too much swallows hope. To love deeply risks great pain with loss, but to favor distance from another as protection against such loss risks unending loneliness. Fear, of course, lay at the core of my experience of Erik's accident. Fear of the unknown, fear of love, and fear of no love. Fear of unending grief and fear of dashed hopes.

In short, Erik's accident resides in my very composition. Even fifteen years later, I confront emotions rooted in that early experience. The accident as omen carries both portent and promise. It holds simultaneously both my darkest memories and my most solid foundation. It contains both darkness and light. The day I returned to school after the accident I had a strong emotion that has stuck with me ever since. I felt that no one in the world could ever truly appreciate what I was experiencing. I grew to understand that this tragedy was mine; I owned it in a way no one else could. My appreciation of life and the darkness and complexity it held became vitally important. In fact, I became deeply committed to a very solemn and undying optimism that formed the foundation of my identity.

I cannot accept a singular perspective on the world; I see and understand a delicate balance between love and hate. I have hated the accident, for it simultaneously took away the brother I knew and loved and created a brother different from the one I was familiar with. He was an impostor in my young eyes. How could I, as a thirteen-year-old, explain to others why Erik was so different from me? This was a new brother, and the old one was gone.

I now recognize the ways in which Erik became idealized to me; his accident was for all of us a small death that froze in time my perceptions of who he had been. It was impossible to grieve for this in light of the comatose but breathing and living creature before me. As I began to understand the complexity of my emotions, I began to release my binding assumptions of "normalcy." There is no such thing as a "normal" life, one which a person gets back after any given experience. We limit ourselves and one another by such constrictive assumptions and expectations.

The family unit itself—whatever form it takes—can be understood as an organism, each member influencing the others. Perhaps we balance each other's energies in harmony. As an organism, the family might be analogous to the human brain. If injury to the brain produces loss or impairment of function in one area, other pathways may be created, or one can compensate through new strategies or by strengthening other senses. It is helpful for me to imagine the family as one body with multiple capacities, perspectives, and responses. With injury and loss or new life to a family come new responses, reassigned capabilities, and revised roles for each member of the unit. To have undying faith in some frozen view of "normalcy" is to live in constant fear of transformation.

Erik's affliction, and our experimentation with narration and narratives in response to his and our need to make meaning from this event, led me to reconsider selfhood and to rethink the humanist discourse in which a person appears as the primary mover or central actor in his life story. Instead, I learned to see through absence and nonaction, or what is not, to hidden presence, or that which might be called forth through caring interactions. Gropingly, our experiments with stories challenged the privilege granted to the scientific-medical worldview by contributing fragments of poetry, fiction, philosophy, and insights from spiritual traditions and by inquiring into the relationship between language and power. Gradually, by listening with all our senses as well as our intellects, we began to entertain and to perceive the story-dependent quality of the body-brain organism itself. In recounting these experiments I assume, as David Morris does in writing about the history and interpretation of pain, that a conversation between medical professionals and writers will expand our understanding of brain injury and the possibilities for reconstructing the self.[13] In short, our journey with brain injury suggests the therapeutic potential of narratives not simply for individuals with traumatic brain injury but also for those who, by relationship or professional choice, assist them to survive and to reconstruct their lives and for a culture needing to perceive differently or to enlarge its own story about selfhood and the values embodied in that story.

The space that traumatic brain injury opened for us was the hidden dimension of our true condition—our vulnerability as human beings and the utterly relational character of selfhood. We entered this space by force, not by choice, with Erik's temporary eviction from his self house and from his culture. In this space of anxious waiting and intensive labor, "costing not less than everything" we previously thought we knew and understood, I learned that second births are necessary not only for those who lose a former sense of self through traumatic brain injury.[14] Choosing to be answerable with one's own life "for everyone else and everything" also calls for a second birth, a radical turn toward those conditions or characteristics in ourselves and others that are hidden from view.

By themselves, those afflicted with brain injuries initially cannot find beginnings in endings nor generally see their own lives as creative works. And they, like other people, cannot alone become answerable to their experience. To know ourselves as unified, and dynamic, subjects and objects is a capacity acquired through relationship. Only through active and creative interactions with those who are able to embrace and willing to experiment with disintegration, and who imagine that their responsiveness to their own unity may make more likely the reconstruction of those who have been unhoused, can the brain injured and the uninjured approach answerability. By assisting in the tedious sorting of bits and scraps of a former self, by patiently helping to lay the fragments out on bare boards, by carefully witnessing and supporting the arrangement of old pieces into a new narrative, the uninjured and the injured together can prepare for the second birth into the house of relational Being.

Epilogue

Crossing the Threshold

The Navajo say:	Those who tell the stories rule the world.
But a story that is told	is not the story enacted.
A cold wind played	outside our house one
February night in 1995	as the family sat inside
again around	the kitchen table.
When I finished reading	the draft of chapter one,
a tale familiar	from frequent tellings, Erik said,
"You must go on, for until	you finish writing, I will not be finished."
You and I, he said.	I and he? I thought.
Neither will be finished	till the story be told out,
till *he* becomes	a *you* again.
I pondered puzzled:	how writing his story
could complete him.	Perhaps he meant
he could not be	himself unless I wrote
him to the present.	Was it an ending
or release	he called for?
Did I need to	write him across *his* gaps—
or were the gaps	now more *mine* than his,
a teller and the tale	seeking communion with the told?

In 1995 Erik initially encouraged me to continue writing the story of his reconstruction, for he hoped others in similar circumstances might find help and solace from the telling. I believe that the idea that he would not be finished until I completed the writing expressed his longing to be released from changes and losses that felt like death and from the judgments often assigned to those afflicted with acquired brain injuries.

Five years later, in the spring of 2000, I gave Erik my completed manuscript of his reconstructed life to read. I waited. When he telephoned two weeks later, I was surprised to hear him say, "Well, Mom, I've finished the book." Silence. "That's good," I said. Then he began to express dismay, saying clearly that the stories that are told may not be the story that is enacted.

"Mom, this book treats me like an object. It is very disempowering. Oh, it may empower the family, but it certainly disempowers me." Stunned, but also listening in the spaces between his words, I wanted to know more. "Can you explain or illustrate what you mean?" I asked. "Well, the book doesn't talk about me." Incredulous, I wondered wordlessly about whom he thought I had written. He continued, "You know, the book makes me sound like I'm still crazy. Though you don't intend it, you're destroying my life with this book. This story may inadvertently give others a basis to judge me inaccurately in the present or to treat me with prejudice. Is there any reason to go beyond high school?"

"Why would you want me to stop the story at high school when so many changes and significant growth continued well beyond high school?" I asked. He offered two related reasons. First, to contain his struggles and disorientations to high school, which was by now a safe distance in the past, would protect his present, forward-moving life. Second, he feared that acquaintances and colleagues who have not known his history now might regard him differently with this information. His hesitancies resounded in me, for indeed my own ambivalence about choosing vulnerability for the entire family, and for many others who have been important to Erik's reconstruction, had protracted the writing process. We discussed at length the risks associated with vulnerability, as he vacillated between self-protection and disclosure.

Suddenly in the midst of this discussion about transparency he referred me to a passage in the manuscript where I described his disintegration, saying that he didn't act like our son. "Mom, is this still a question for you and Dad? How am I or am I not your son?" I was stung by his question. Although he was never not our son, the son we knew is not the son we know. I began to perceive that he was asking if I could see him beneath the terms I used to describe his behaviors and conditions. How profound that question is for anyone who suffers an injury or illness that affects identity. As we talked on, I understood that he wanted to know if we still viewed him as a collection of shattered pieces, or if we knew and loved him as a whole spirit-being called our son. His questions were the hardest any reader of the manuscript had raised, but the fact that Erik could conceptually and emotionally pose them bore witness to this fact: he had recovered. He merely questioned whether we fathomed that he is now fully living his life. His questions belong with the usually unarticulated ones that each of us lives daily: Who am I to you? Do you see me in parts or in whole? Through your eyes or mine? How am I myself because of the ways you see and relate to me?

Erik challenged my describing his life narrative as interrupted. "Mom, what was interrupted were your preconceived ideas of what my life was or would be. This was my life, my narrative." Apparently to Erik, who had lived the disintegration when he could not speak about it, the past and the present, former abilities and altered ones, were all one fabric. Speaking as the enacter of his story, he continued to explain, "The more a person who has suffered a brain injury goes over the preconceived notion of himself, his story, the more depressed he is liable to get. If I had held the former self out in front of me, I would have given up or gotten depressed."

As I had continued writing watching closely, looking backward, Erik proceeded living forward, becoming author of a more important sort. He designed a second career, plotted job searches independently, and found fine employment among books as a servant to the public. Simultaneously he began to weave his life through love with a young woman, whom he married. And in July 1999 they brought forth new life—a daughter, grand and beautiful. Living through his woundedness, Erik sees continuity in his life. Looking backward as parents, we have wrestled with discontinuities.

In several lengthy phone conversations over three days, author as enacter confronted author as teller. I listened attentively, for I suspected that Erik and I were witnessing a profound integration—or perhaps several integrations. Erik had read the manuscript closely and had meticulously identified passages about which he had questions or recommendations for emphasis or word changes. Of all those who have carefully read versions of this manuscript, Erik's reading was indeed the most remarkable and valuable. His attention to my efforts to describe the reshaping of his shattered life revealed that he had achieved a seamless mental and emotional integration. Furthermore, by responding from within the enacted story, he set in bold relief the book's purpose: to show that although any told story is not the enacted story, that which is told becomes the "reality" that people see and to which they react. Robert and Sonia and I had been bound together in this intimate struggle with death and life, yet we had our stories and he his.

Erik's own thoughtful response to the manuscript prompted important revisions that have made the book infinitely richer and more honest. His acute awareness of the needs and feelings of those confronted with disabling conditions, unexpected injury, or prolonged illness invites author-teller and reader to consider the multiple dimensions of his life—and the life of anyone who suffers an identity-altering injury or illness—and how it may be perceived. It illuminates the distinction between the story he has enacted and continues to live and the one I have perceived and told as a participant-observer of his efforts to reconstruct self-identity. His dismay that in telling his story I and the reader might lose sight of him, the one who lives within that which is told, not only reveals his sensitivity to partial truth and how it can disempower but also implicitly acknowledges that every act of interpretation threatens misrepresentation. Erik's reactions, instead of diminishing the story about his reconstruction process, brought us as adult child and parent into healthy dialogue. Both as storyteller and parent, I need his criticisms and support to make genuine knowing possible. His ability to tell and mine to listen—the capacity of each to give to the other what each needs—signals the psychological maturation that the accident and reconstruction process required of all of us.

When Erik asked if we could see *him* amidst all his changes and the re-storying of his life, he was not concerned with invisibility. Rather, he posed a more profound double observation about writing in general: first, that the told story is not the enacted story, and, second, that personal prejudices and insecurities can shape perceptions, leading people to abstract from told or enacted stories only self-selected pieces. Erik was far less fearful of disclosure than that others—the readers of the book—might misuse what is told or would fail to see through to the fullness of truth.

No one could have more fitting closing words than Erik. Personally acquainted with prolonged silence and the long struggle to the light, Erik's experience calls us individually and collectively toward personal and social maturation. His journey of reconstruction suggests that selective perception and prejudices sustained by partial or narrow stories discriminate unfairly against recovery or the reconstruction of a new being. Rather than closing the breach between things that are dying and those waiting to be born anew, partial stories widen and deepen such divides.

With Erik we have learned, as have other families confronted with traumatic brain injury, that bridging the gaps created by brain injury requires enormous effort. No partial story nor single story type is adequate for the reconstruction of self-identity. Rather, varieties of stories with a broad array of narrators are necessary to support our psychological work and collective awakening to our own relational being. Stories that enlarge, complicate, and even contradict bring us into relationship, protect us from fragmentary stories intended to control or manipulate, and provide a basis to overcome rather than reinforce prejudice; they anchor without enchaining. Relational telling—from multiple voices, visions, and locations—gives stories therapeutic potential by bringing enactment and telling closer together. Telling that respects the feeling basis of thought and explores the biological ground of perception nourishes the imagination of both teller and hearer, making them knower and known to themselves and others and participants in a natural order alive with polyphonic communication. Stories that incarnate mutual support and love empower and heal.

Erik has done his part in overcoming the rift in his being produced by brain injury. Two questions remain. Does his experience enable us to recognize all brokenness and disabilities as belonging to us? Will we choose to reach across the gaps that occur in us and in others, live in the cracks of the unknown, and cross the threshold from oblivion toward relational being? This book is, in the end, dedicated to this challenge and invitation.

Acknowledgments

I have written this book to bear grateful witness to the resiliency of the human being and to the sacred web of Being that holds and nourishes all life. Arising from silence, the book has been called forth by a host of people, known and unknown to me. Those who surrounded Erik and our family with acts of care, from highly skilled medical and rehabilitation services to invisible prayers, have made it possible for us to live in the gaps created by the unexpected intrusion of traumatic brain injury. I trust that both those named in the preceding pages as well as those acknowledged simply by their actions will understand the debt I feel and that their services rendered to assist the reconstruction of one young man's life will inspire others to do likewise. I am especially grateful for the memory of my sister, Sharon Knechel, and of Michael Cox, whose acts—Sharon through her devotion, wit, and indefatigable belief in Erik, and Mike through his courageous ability to hold fast to hope with Erik even in his own suffering and dying—have left imperishable imprints on our lives.

As the vision for this book began to take form in my mind, several people encouraged and helped me define the directions it might take. I gratefully include Arthur Kleinman, George Howard, Al Neiman,

Stephen Fredman, Anne Harrington, Janice Radway, Jean Lee, John Winslade, Gerald Monk, and Judith Kelleher. James Langford and Alice Calaprice offered invaluable professional guidance on publication matters. Behind these named stand the unnamed who have themselves also sustained brain injuries and their families. Conversations with them in hospitals, in head injury groups, in halfway houses, and in their homes have informed this work and remind me that there is yet more to tell.

In bringing forth a highly personal text within an academic profession, I benefited exceedingly from the support of friends and colleagues whose careful reading of the manuscript and wise editorial suggestions made the prose clearer. To Kathy Royer, Barbara Turpin, Jane Doering, Bernard Doering, Carol Schaal, Marcia Lemay, and Michael Driscoll I express my sincere appreciation. Three other individuals deserve special recognition for their part in letting the story speak. Arthur Frank, whose own extensive work on illness narratives, read the manuscript with keen sensitivity for giving voice to the afflicted. His recommendations have significantly strengthened the narrative. Reading with knowledge of and attentiveness to the tremendous challenges traumatic brain injury poses, Paul Macellari recommended subtle but important changes in emphasis and permitted me to see Erik through an outsider's eyes and experience. Finally, I am indebted to my editor, Stanley Holwitz, first for his commitment to this book, and second for his persistent conviction to help it communicate with multiple audiences. The final stages of this project have been made immeasurably easier by Dore Brown's sensitive oversight of the book's production and by Marian Olivas's meticulous attention to editorial details.

Completing this project would have been far more difficult without assistance from the Institute for Scholarship in the Liberal Arts at the University of Notre Dame, from the dean of the College of Arts and Letters, Mark Roche, from Maureen Jones, who ably handled administrative details, from my student research assistant, Kim Krug, who collected library resources and helped to proofread an early draft, and from

Cheryl Reed, who patiently tolerated my experimentation with formats and carefully typed numerous drafts.

No one knows this book better than those to whom it is dedicated. Although it can never fully convey the way each of them experienced the events described here, Robert's, Erik's, and Sonia's courage to live in the gaps, their faith that by trudging the gaps together we might be guided to fuller awareness, and their repeated forgiveness when any of us leaned toward giving up daily embodied the transformative power of love. I offer them, and the three new beings of hope, my abiding love and gratitude.

Notes

Threshold 1. The Impact of Vulnerability

1. The Glasgow Coma Scale was developed by the Neurosciences Department of Glasgow University in 1974. The lowest total mark on the scale is 3; the highest total mark is 15. The scale is useful not simply for estimating the severity of the brain injury but also for measuring the lightening of a coma. Patients with total scores of 3, 4, or 5 are considered to have very severe brain injuries. Those with scores of 6, 7, or 8 have a severe brain injury. Patients with a rating of 9 or higher may be out of coma but still suffer effects of brain injury. See E. A. Freeman, *The Catastrophe of Coma: A Way Back* (Australia/New Zealand: David Bateman, 1987), 34–40.

Threshold 3. Uncertain Deliveries

1. William Winslade, *Confronting Traumatic Brain Injury: Devastation, Hope, and Healing* (New Haven: Yale University Press, 1998), 30.
2. Winslade, *Confronting Traumatic Brain Injury*, 31.
3. Winslade, *Confronting Traumatic Brain Injury*, 31.

Threshold 4. Becoming Again

1. M. Merleau-Ponty, *Phenomenology of Perception*, trans. Colin Smith (London: Routledge, 1992), 9.

2. David Abram, *The Spell of the Sensuous: Perception and Language in a More-Than-Human World* (New York: Pantheon Books, 1996).

3. Charles Dickens, "Night Walks," in *Charles Dickens: Selected Journalism 1850–1870* (New York: Penguin Books, 1997), 73 and 77.

4. Antonio R. Damasio, *The Feeling of What Happens: Body and Emotion in the Making of Consciousness* (New York: Harcourt Brace & Co., 1999).

5. Augustine, *The Confessions of Saint Augustine*, trans. Edward B. Pusey (New York: Pocket Books, Inc., 1956), 1:8.

6. T. S. Eliot, "Ash Wednesday," in *Collected Poems 1909–1962* (New York: Harcourt, Brace & World, 1983), 86.

7. See Damasio, *The Feeling of What Happens*, chapters 6 and 7, for elaboration of core and extended consciousness.

Threshold 5. The Scattered Self

1. In *The Archaeology of Knowledge* and *The Order of Things* Foucault discusses at length how history, narratively presented, obscures the real events by ignoring disintegrating movements or forces in the "story of civilization" and becomes a form of repression. See Richard Poirier's discussion of Foucault's ideas in his chapter "Writing Off the Self" in *The Renewal of Literature: Emersonian Reflections* (New York: Random House, 1987), 187.

2. *The Wishing Bone Cycle: Narrative Poems from the Swampy Cree Indians*, gathered and trans. Howard A. Norman (Santa Barbara: Ross-Erickson Publishing, 1972), 5.

3. See Ellen Basso, "The Trickster's Scattered Self," *Anthropological Linguistics* 30 (1988): 3–4, 292–318, for a discussion of tricksters as narrativized selves.

4. Damasio, *The Feeling of What Happens*, 191.

5. Arthur W. Frank, *The Wounded Storyteller: Body, Illness, and Ethics* (Chicago: University of Chicago Press, 1995).

6. Martin Heidegger, *Basic Writings from Being and Time (1927) to The Task of Thinking (1964)* (New York: Harper & Row Publishers, 1977), 193–242.

7. Frank R. Wilson, *The Hand: How Its Use Shapes the Brain, Language, and Human Culture* (New York: Vintage Books, 1998), 277, 59.

8. John Dewey, *How We Think* (New York: Prometheus Books, 1991), 11.

9. Dewey, *How We Think*, 29.

10. Dewey, *How We Think,* 30.

11. Antonio R. Damasio, *Descartes' Error: Emotion, Reason, and the Human Brain* (New York: Avon Books, 1994), 247.

12. "The Infinite Mind: Psychosis," interview of Charles Jennings on *The Infinite Mind,* host Fred Goodwin, National Public Radio, 21 Feb. 2000.

Threshold 6. Improvisational Selves

1. Odie L. Bracy, "Cognitive Functioning and Rehabilitation," *The Journal of Cognitive Rehabilitation* 12, no. 2 (1994): 14.

2. See Bracy, "Cognitive Functioning and Rehabilitation," for a discussion of the executive skills.

3. Psychological evaluation for Erik Johansen, Child Development and Rehabilitation, Children's Seashore House and the Children's Hospital of Philadelphia, unpublished record, 30 June 1987, 4.

4. Odie L. Bracy, "Cognitive Rehabilitation: A Process Approach," *Cognitive Rehabilitation* 4, no. 2 (1986), 11.

5. Bracy, "Cognitive Functioning and Rehabilitation," 16.

6. Damasio, *The Feeling of What Happens*, 142.

7. Kabir, *The Kabir Book: Forty-four of the Ecstatic Poems of Kabir,* versions by Robert Bly (Boston: Beacon Press, 1977), 11.

Threshold 7. Accepting Vulnerability

1. T. S. Eliot, "Little Gidding," from *Four Quartets* (New York: Harcourt Brace & Co., 1971), 58.

2. Julia Kristeva, *Desire in Language: A Semiotic Approach to Literature and Art,* ed. Leon S. Roudiez, trans. Thomas Gora, Alice Jardine, and Leon S. Roudiez (New York: Columbia University Press, 1980), 25.

3. Statistics from the Brain Injury Association and the Centers for Disease Control show that every fifteen seconds one person in the United States sustains a brain injury, that every year 373,000 persons are hospitalized with traumatic brain injury and survive, and that males between fourteen and twenty-four years of age are at highest risk, followed by infants and the elderly.

4. Kristeva, *Desire in Language*, 23.

5. Kristeva, *Desire in Language*, 6.

6. Kristeva, *Desire in Language*, 6–7.

7. Nel Noddings, *Caring: A Feminine Approach to Ethics and Moral Education* (Berkeley and Los Angeles: University of California Press, 1984), 4–5. See also Michael Bérubé, *Life as We Know It: A Father, a Family, and an Exceptional Child* (New York: Vintage Books, 1996), 241–248, for his discussion of reciprocity as described by Jürgen Habermas and John Rawls.

8. Michael Katz, Nel Noddings, and Kenneth Strike, eds., *Justice and Caring: The Search for Common Ground in Education* (New York: Teachers College Press, 1999), 16.

9. Fyodor Dostoevsky, *The Brothers Karamazov,* trans. Andrew H. MacAndrew (1860; New York: Bantam Books, 1981), 347.

10. M. M. Bakhtin, *Art and Answerability: Early Philosophical Essays,* ed. and trans. Michael Holquist and Vadim Liapunov (Austin: University of Texas Press, 1990), 1.

11. Bérubé, *Life as We Know It*, 248.

12. Bérubé, *Life as We Know It*, 241.

13. David Morris, *The Culture of Pain* (Berkeley and Los Angeles: University of California Press, 1991).

14. Eliot, "Little Gidding," 59.

Bibliography

Abram, David. *The Spell of the Sensuous: Perception and Language in a More-Than-Human World.* New York: Pantheon Books, 1996.

Augustine. *The Confessions of St. Augustine.* Trans. Edward B. Pusey. New York: Pockct Books, Inc., 1956.

Bakhtin, M. M. *Art and Answerability: Early Philosophical Essays.* Ed. and trans. Michael Holquist and Vadim Liapunov. Austin: University of Texas Press, 1990.

————. *The Dialogic Imagination.* Ed. Michael Holquist. Trans. Caryl Emerson and Michael Holquist. Austin: University of Texas Press, 1981.

Basso, Ellen. "The Trickster's Scattered Self." *Anthropological Linguistics* 30 (1988): 3–4, 292–318.

Bérubé, Michael. *Life as We Know It: A Father, a Family, and an Exceptional Child.* New York: Vintage Books, 1996.

Bracy, Odie L. "Cognitive Functioning and Rehabilitation." *The Journal of Cognitive Rehabilitation* 12, no. 2 (1994): 12–16.

————. "Cognitive Rehabilitation: A Process Approach." *Cognitive Rehabilitation* 4, no. 2 (1986): 10–17.

Bruner, Jerome. *Acts of Meaning.* Cambridge, Mass.: Harvard University Press, 1990.

————. *Actual Minds, Possible Worlds.* Cambridge, Mass.: Harvard University Press, 1986.

Chaney, Norman. *Six Images of Human Nature.* Englewood Cliffs, N.J.: Prentice Hall, 1990.

Chodorow, Nancy J. *The Power of Feelings: Personal Meaning in Psychoanalysis, Gender, and Culture.* New Haven, Conn.: Yale University Press, 1999.

Cortazzi, Martin. *Narrative Analysis.* London: The Falsner Press, 1993.

Crosby, John F. *The Selfhood of the Human Person.* Washington, D.C.: The Catholic University Press of America, 1996.

Damasio, Antonio R. *Descartes' Error: Emotion, Reason, and the Human Brain.* New York: Avon Books, 1994.

———. *The Feeling of What Happens: Body and Emotion in the Making of Consciousness.* New York: Harcourt Brace & Co., 1999.

Dennett, D. C. *Consciousness Explained.* New York: Little Brown, 1991.

Dewey, John. *How We Think.* 1910; reprint Amherst: Prometheus Books, 1991.

Dickens, Charles. "Night Walks." In *Charles Dickens: Selected Journalism 1850–1870.* New York: Penguin Books, 1997.

Dostoevsky, Fyodor. *The Brothers Karamazov.* Trans. Andrew H. MacAndrew. 1860; reprint New York: Bantam Books, 1981.

Dudai, Y. *The Neurobiology of Memory: Concepts, Findings, Trends.* New York: Oxford University Press, 1989.

Eliot, T. S. *Collected Poems 1909–1962.* 1963; reprint New York: Harcourt, Brace & World, 1983.

———. *Four Quartets.* 1943; reprint New York: Harcourt Brace & Co., 1971.

Ellis, Ralph. *An Ontology of Consciousness.* Boston: Martinus Nijhoff Publishers, 1986.

Epston, David, Kathie Crocket, Gerald Monk, and John Winslade, eds. *Narrative Therapy in Practice: The Archaeology of Hope.* San Francisco: Jossey-Bass Publishers, 1997.

Franck, Frederick. *To Be Human against All Odds.* Berkeley, Calif.: Asian Humanities Press, 1991.

Frank, Arthur W. *At the Will of the Body.* New York: Houghton Mifflin, 1991.

———. *The Wounded Storyteller: Body, Illness, and Ethics.* Chicago: University of Chicago Press, 1995.

Freeman, E. A. *The Catastrophe of Coma: A Way Back.* Australia/New Zealand: David Bateman, 1987.

Gardner, Harold. *Frames of Mind: The Theory of Multiple Intelligences.* New York: Basic Books, 1983.

Genette, Gérard. *Narrative Discourse: An Essay on Method.* Trans. Jane E. Lewin. Ithaca, N.Y.: Cornell University Press, 1980.

Gergen, Kenneth. "Technology and the Self: From the Essential to the Sublime." In *Constructing the Self in a Mediated World.* Ed. Debra Grodin and Thomas R. Lindlof. Thousand Oaks, Calif.: Sage Publications, 1996.

Gergen, Kenneth J., and Mary M. Gergen, eds. *Historical Social Psychology.* Hillsdale: Lawrence Erlbaum Associates, 1984.

Girard, René. *Deceit, Desire, and the Novel: Self and Other in Literary Structure.* Trans. Yvonne Freccero. Baltimore: Johns Hopkins University Press, 1961.

Goethals, George R., and Jaine Strauss, eds. *The Self: Interdisciplinary Approaches.* New York: Springer-Verlag, 1991.

Grossman, Marshall. "The Subject of Narrative and the Rhetoric of Self." *Papers on Language and Literature* 18, no. 4 (1982): 398–415.

Harvey, Robert L. *Neural Network Principles.* Englewood Cliffs, N.J.: Prentice Hall, 1994.

Heidegger, Martin. *Basic Writings from Being and Time (1927) to The Task of Thinking (1964).* New York: Harper & Row Publishers, 1977.

Hertzfeld, Michael. *The Poetics of Manhood: Contest and Identity in a Cretan Mountain Village.* Princeton, N.J.: Princeton University Press, 1985.

Johnson, M. *The Bodily Basis of Meaning, Imagination, and Reason.* Chicago: University of Chicago Press, 1987.

Kabir. *The Kabir Book: Forty-four of the Ecstatic Poems of Kabir.* Versions by Robert Bly. Boston: Beacon Press, 1977.

Katz, Michael, Nel Noddings, and Kenneth A. Strike, eds. *Justice and Caring: The Search for Common Ground in Education.* New York: Teachers College Press, 1999.

Kerby, Anthony Paul. *Narrative and the Self.* Bloomington: Indiana University Press, 1991.

Kleinman, Arthur. *The Illness Narratives: Suffering, Healing and the Human Condition.* New York: Basic Books, 1988.

Komesaroff, Paul A. *Troubled Bodies: Critical Perspectives on Postmodernism, Medical Ethics, and the Body.* Durham, N.C.: Duke University Press, 1995.

Kotulak, Ronald. *Inside the Brain: Revolutionary Discoveries of How the Mind Works.* Kansas City: Andrews and McMeel, 1996.

Kristeva, Julia. *Desire in Language: A Semiotic Approach to Literature and Art.*

Ed. Leon S. Roudiez. Trans. Thomas Gora, Alice Jardine, and Leon S. Roudiez. New York: Columbia University Press, 1980.

Linde, Charlotte. *Life Stories: The Creation of Coherence.* New York: Oxford University Press, 1993.

Llinas, Rodolfo R., ed. *The Biology of the Brain: From Neurons to Networks.* New York: W.H. Freeman & Co., 1989.

Luria, A. R. *Restoration of Function after Brain Injury.* Trans. Basil Haigh. Ed. O. L. Zanqwill. New York: Macmillan, 1963.

———. *The Working Brain: An Introduction to Neuropsychology.* Trans. Basil Haigh. New York: Basic Books, 1973.

Merleau-Ponty, M. *Phenomenology of Perception.* Trans. Colin Smith. London: Routledge, 1992.

Miller, Nancy K., ed. *The Poetics of Gender.* New York: Columbia University Press, 1986.

Mira-Mira, Jose, and Roberto Moreno-Diaz, eds. *Brain Processes, Theories and Models: An International Conference in Honor of W. S. McCulloch 25 Years after His Death.* Cambridge, Mass.: Massachusetts Institute of Technology, 1996.

Mitchell, W. J. T. *On Narrative.* Chicago: University of Chicago Press, 1980.

Morris, David. *The Culture of Pain.* Berkeley and Los Angeles: University of California Press, 1991.

Nelson, Hilde Lindemann, ed. *Stories and Their Limits.* New York: Routledge, 1997.

Nochi, Masahiro. "'Loss of Self' in the Narratives of People with Traumatic Brain Injuries: A Qualitative Analysis." *Social Science and Medicine* 46, no. 7 (1998): 869–878.

Noddings, Nel. *Caring: A Feminine Approach to Ethics and Moral Education.* Berkeley and Los Angeles: University of California Press, 1984.

Ornstein, Robert. *The Psychology of Consciousness.* New York: Viking Penguin, 1973.

Poirier, Richard. *The Renewal of Literature: Emersonian Reflections.* New York: Random House, 1987.

Ramachandran, V. A., and Sandra Blakeslee. *Phantoms in the Brain: Probing the Mysteries of the Human Mind.* New York: William Morrow, 1998.

Roberts, Glenn, and Jeremy Holmes. *Healing Stories: Narrative in Psychiatry and Psychotherapy.* New York: Oxford University Press, 1999.

Rutter, M., and M. Rutter. *Developing Minds: Challenge and Continuity across the Lifespan*. New York: Basic Books, 1993.

Ryan, Marie-Laure. *Possible Worlds, Artificial Intelligence, and Narrative Theory*. Bloomington: Indiana University Press, 1991.

Scarry, Elaine. *The Body in Pain: The Making and Unmaking of the World*. New York: Oxford University Press, 1985.

Searle, J. R. *The Rediscovery of Mind*. Cambridge, Mass.: Bradford Books, MIT Press, 1992.

Shafer, Roy. *Retelling a Life: Narration and Dialogue in Psychoanalysis*. New York: Basic Books, 1992.

Taylor, Charles. *Sources of the Self: The Making of Modern Identity*. Cambridge, Mass.: Harvard University Press, 1989.

Todorov, Tzvetan. *Mikhail Bakhtin: The Dialogical Principle* Trans Wlad Godzich. Minneapolis: University of Minnesota Press, 1984.

White, Michael, and David Epston. *Narrative Means to Therapeutic Ends*. New York: W. W. Norton & Company, 1990.

Wilson, Frank R. *The Hand: How Its Use Shapes the Brain, Language, and Human Culture*. New York: Vintage Books, 1998.

Winslade, William. *Confronting Traumatic Brain Injury: Devastation, Hope, and Healing*. New Haven, Conn.: Yale University Press, 1998.

The Wishing Bone Cycle: Narrative Poems from the Swampy Cree Indians. Gathered and trans. Howard A. Norman. Santa Barbara: Ross-Erickson Publishing, 1972.

Index

Indexer: Patricia Deminna
Compositor: Integrated Composition Systems
Text: 11/15 Granjon
Display: Granjon
Printer and binder: Haddon Craftsmen